My Lupus, My Problem

A Love-Hate Story

Johnny Thomas

Dedication

To everyone fighting lupus or any chronic illness that nobody can see.

To everyone who's been told "you don't look sick" when you're dying inside.

To everyone who wanted to give up but kept going anyway.

This book is for you.

You are not alone. You are a warrior.

Stay in the fight. You're here for a reason.

Just like me.

Acknowledgement

First, I got to thank God. For keeping me here. For giving me strength when I had none left. For turning my pain into my purpose.

To my rheumatologists. You became my family. You treated me with respect. You believed me. You fought for me. Thank you.

To my wound care team. You see my wounds every week and you treat me with kindness. You never made me feel like a burden. Thank you for caring.

To my fiancée. Through everything. Through the blood, the pain, the hospital visits. When I tried to push you away, you stayed. You are my angel. Thank you for loving me. Lupus and all.

To myself. Yeah, I'm thanking myself too. Because I fought when everyone said I wouldn't make it. I was born too small to survive. But I'm still here. Still fighting. Thank you, Johnny, for not giving up.

And to everyone reading this. Thank you for hearing my story. Thank you for caring about people like me.

Stay in the fight. Keep going.

You're here for a reason.

Contents

Dedication iii

Acknowledgement iv

Chapter 1 The Spice of My Life and Finding My Right Flavor to Keep My Faith Strong................................ 1

Chapter 2 Getting Through Challenges That Tried to Kill My Faith 15

Chapter 3 Cooking: The Blessing in My Life.............. 26

Chapter 4 Recreating Myself After Lupus Changed My Work Life.. 37

Chapter 5 Pulling All My Strength to Keep My Journey Moving 52

Chapter 6 Mastering My Financial Issues.................... 65

Chapter 7 The Music That Got Me Through Most of These Challenges in My Life 84

Chapter 8: How I Locked Down My Community With My Weekend Breakfast and Dinners 104

Chapter 9 How I Ignore the Negativity to Keep A Positive Mindset 126

Chapter 10 How I Had to Learn to Have Patience With All Things in My Life................................... 142

Chapter 11 Mastering the Craft I Love Most in Life 155

Chapter 12 From A Normal Life to A Life Living With Lupus.. 173

Chapter 13 A Couple of Dreams I Had Before I Got Lupus.. 196

Chapter 14 How I Spiritually Nourish My Soul 216

Chapter 15 Did God Bless Me with Lupus to Make Me A Wiser Person?.. 244

Chapter 16 Turning My Pain Into A Purpose 275

Chapter 17 The Shocking News of My Community .. 300

Chapter 18 The Affections of a Favorite Pet 324

Chapter 19 The Amazing Effects of Having That Special One in Your Life 359

Chapter 20 The Poem of My Life with Lupus 377

Chapter 1
The Spice of My Life and Finding My Right Flavor to Keep My Faith Strong

So let me stir you away into the world of spices that become magical flavors. Ha ha, yes, I am like a magical magician in the kitchen, known as the Master Barber Chef Doctor. I can make a meal that captures the mind of anyone internationally, and I can give you a Master Barber full-service grooming treatment that will transform your entire life! Your lifestyle will remain booming forever, no matter what time or kind of weather. Once my ingredients enter your life, you will start feeling right in the way you want and deserve.

My spiritual life before lupus was what I thought was average, normal even. I was a part of a lot of churches and a certain group of friends. We all played the same sports: boxing and football. We all worked at the same employment facility. I thought everything about myself was like any other normal kid transitioning from teenager to young adult. I always had strong faith in myself that I would have a successful future rather than a corrupt one. I constantly tried to upgrade my lifestyle as time went on, trying to keep updated with most of my friends who had plans for the future. I never thought of anything other than to keep striving to do good in my life.

One of my goals, dreams, and passions is to help many suffering and struggling souls find a much more powerful way, a clearer path to a successful future. Whether God plans for us to meet one day in person or you connect with me through my own experiences that I've written in this book, I want to make a difference. As me and my lupus travel through this life journey together, we refuse to let trials and tribulations get in our way or stop us from achieving and reaching our goals in life.

My cooking comes from my mother and grandmother. Growing up in the '70s, I was always amazed, always wondering how they got the food to taste so delicious. Sometimes I even compared my mom's cooking to my grandmother's cooking, but it was too hard to choose because they both cooked so well.

When they weren't around (if they were at work or running some errands), I'd try to surprise my mom by cooking something up. I first started by learning how to bake bread and make homemade cakes from scratch using that old all-purpose flour. I'd add eggs and milk and sugar with butter to make the cakes. And when I made the bread, I used flour with salt, butter, cornstarch, and one egg for extra taste. I just thought adding eggs was always a must for any baking-type dish.

And it was so fun and felt so good to see that I could actually do this. When I let my friends and some family members try what I made, they were amazed and surprised it came out not just okay, but really good. It gave me confidence to get into cooking more and more. And my cooking journey started from there.

I can't begin to tell you how tired me and my lupus are, so tired of hearing time after time from the people in this world. And I'm talking about people who are supposed to be professionals, all the way down to ordinary everyday people who see everyday life challenges with an illness that God blesses His special angels with. When I look back to when I was growing up, I think about how I was being brought up and couldn't believe I thought some of that was normal and okay. This is one of the reasons why I truly believe God blessed me to have lupus in my life. It's like having an angel who watches over me, who helps me secure every step I take to improve my lifestyle. Lupus guides me on how I should be living, how I should be eating, and the way I should be thinking at all times. It's backup security in my life, keeping me on the right path.

And yes, I believe a lot of people can relate to what I'm talking about. When you grow up admiring the wrong role models, you make many wrong choices in life. Even if you have good parents and the best school teachers, you waste time around the wrong people, the wrong food, and the wrong music, you will lose it. You'll lose yourself from being on the right track in life.

As time went on in my cooking journey, I started trying out different fancy stuff, like high-class cooking. For some reason I was always a fan of seafood! I used to hear my older relatives always talking about how they loved to eat fish, shrimps and lobsters, clams, mussels, and oysters. By the time I started cooking that type of food, I was about 18 or 19 years old.

One of my favorite recipes, one of my favorite dishes, became Fried Red Jamaican Snapper, fried slow in peanut oil with Jamaican bell pepper. I'm also a huge fan of spicy food and seasonings, so this dish was perfect for me. I cook my red snapper with peanut oil, dicing up rainbow sweet peppers along with bell peppers (red, green, and yellow) along with yellow onions and purple onions. I fry the fish until it's lightly brown on both sides, then bake it just a little bit for extra tenderness inside. I make my favorite dumplings smothered in a garlic butter sauce. And in another pot I'll have purple cabbage with slices of carrots and diced up Cajun pepper and butter. For my drink, I top it all off with red beets and carrot juice blended together that I made from scratch. Yes, I'm also a good homemade natural fruits and vegetables juice maker.

That's what I call my very own personal celebration-type dish, the one I prepare for myself when I have a little something on my mind that I'm trying to figure out, my next movements in life. It's such a wonderful, healthy feeling to my mind, body, and soul that I'm able to create a tasty food recipe, my favorite kind of dish. And as time went on, it only got better.

Well, first let me begin with why I consider myself a Master Chef. For many reasons, of course. I study all the foods I eat personally, and I study different cultures around the world. I'm fascinated by foods that tell a story behind the recipe, how each dish was created and how it came to be one of the popular dishes in that particular town or country. I study why I would eat different vegetables on a particular day and time, why I would eat a certain type of meat only once a month, and why I schedule specific times and days of the week to drink certain beverages so I won't become too immune to them.

So just to be clearer on what I'm saying, let me break it down for you. This is just my way of being my own nutritionist and home remedies specialist.

Take Monday, for example. It's the beginning of the week, and everyone knows it's always tough trying to get that day started. Maybe you had a busy weekend that drained your body to where you just want to sleep your Monday away. Your eyes are tired, your joints are sore, and you feel weak and low on energy.

So let me start by saying, for the first three days of the week, I'll eat a small portion of carrots and fresh spinach leaves. I'll mix them in a smoothie for breakfast if I'm running short on time, or I'll chop them up and cook them with egg whites in olive oil. Both methods give you a boost in energy and improve your health system. Carrots are for my eyes, and spinach is for my inflammation, which gives me that pain in my joints that I can't bear sometimes. I'll eat this combination with breakfast, lunch, and dinner for my first three days of the week.

And for the next three days heading into Sunday, I'll eat more fruits and fewer vegetables than I usually would from the beginning of the week. For my breakfast, lunch, and dinner, I'll have blueberries, raspberries, strawberries, a little leafy spinach, and some whole grain toast. And why do I do this in this order? Because I'm preparing myself for a cleansing.

You see, for lunch I'll have a piece of poultry like fish or chicken, and I always eat a small piece of beef or pork once a month. And like I was told, beef and pork aren't all bad for you, but they're not good for you to get carried away with either, especially if you have a special diet you've put yourself on or your doctor has you on. Most mixed berries and leafy greens help break down stubborn foods like beef and pork, helping your digestive system move smoother. When it's time to do a cleansing on Sunday, you'll be starting a whole new healthy eating system routine for the next week.

This is one of the routine recipe programs I shared with some close friends and family members a while back. They made jokes about me, saying, "You're always making all these different styles of dishes and you're always cooking for everyone." They started calling me a Master of different healthy, tasty snacks and food dishes. Eventually, I was just called a Master Chef by the people in my community.

As I was saying before, I was so tired of even telling anyone that I was blessed with lupus, because of the negative things and words that would come out of that individual's mouth. Either they had a cousin or auntie or knew someone who had lupus who passed away, or someone who suffered so terribly they gave up and couldn't do a lot of activities in life like cook, clean, or play sports.

I said to myself, it's because they were surrounded by individuals who are non-believers, people who don't have faith in God to guide them and their lupus in the right path of their life. People who don't know that everything is going to be alright if you believe in your relationship with God, that it's real and strong, and that you, your lupus, and God will become a strong team in your life.

I was always showing off my cooking skills to the women in my life, like when I prepared meals for my daughter and grandkids and for my future wife. To be honest, when I met her, my skills only improved even more because once I saw she doesn't mind a good meal, and she wasn't afraid to show me she enjoys it, it only made me want to cook even more and be much more creative with my cooking. She became my biggest fan and God's blessing of encouragement.

And when I told her about some of the other talents I have besides cooking (I have arts and craft skills, I like to draw different styles of designs, different people, cartoons to real people), I even told her I practiced doing art on my high school friends' haircuts. Yes, I learned how to cut hair a little, then moved to cutting designs into my friends' hair. Like if they liked a certain sneaker, they would tell me to put the symbol and name of that brand of sneaker in their hair.

And those two talents were what I fell in love with, to where I kept up with them for a long period of time, most of my life. Until one day I decided to go get a degree in Master Barbering. And it was a very wonderful new experience to be in a facility surrounded by men and women doing the same thing and having fun while doing it. And to actually graduate with a certified license with my name, "Johnny R. Thomas, Master Barber License." Yes, I felt on top of the world to have completed such a challenging situation.

You have to deal with all walks of life because the barbering school was hands-on, and that comes with a lot of discipline. Different mindsets of different people with different beliefs and attitudes. People all over the world have different styles and different tastes for how they want to look and how they want their image to appear. And of course I satisfied some clients and not others. And to disappoint a client that you want to be proud of your skill, when the cut doesn't come out well, you'll be stunned and can kind of want to give up.

But your mindset, your determination to be strong, to fight and struggle to make yourself hang in there to the finish line of completing your mission that you started, that's a true blessing. And that's what I did. I didn't stop, no matter which client I didn't satisfy. I focused on thinking about the clients I did satisfy, the ones I made happy for that moment, that time of that day. And it took me very far in my faith. My faith just got stronger. And it felt good.

So to hear people I know, people who wish the best for me and want to see me win in life, call me a Master Barber Chef meant so much to me. It meant the world to where I try to always live up to those two titles, that name, that reputation of my life within my journey.

I know I changed my future wife's life through my cooking and haircuts. And I changed three of my closest friends and a few associates from the homeless shelters in New York City. One of the individuals was a man who worked for NBC TV station. Another client was a correction officer in a New York City facility. One was an up-and-rising American supermodel, a young woman at the age of twenty-one years old.

Each person I touched through my craft, whether through a fresh haircut that restored their confidence or a home-cooked meal that reminded them someone cared, each one showed me that God put these talents in my hands for a reason. I wasn't just cutting hair or cooking food. I was changing lives, one person at a time.

One of the first signs I knew something was wrong with my health was the simple fact that after a while, I started to change. My eating habits shifted. My work habits shifted. My interest in doing activities I usually loved just wasn't there anymore. I started losing weight, and I was getting tired very quickly when walking long distances. My skin started being really itchy around my eyes, bringing on a rash around my eyes and face, almost like I was wearing a face mask over my eyes. I was starting to sleep more. My head and all throughout my body felt very sore. I started having arthritis a lot more.

I just knew something wasn't right with me. It was like I was growing older before my time, like I was just aging quickly. Everything I wanted to do, like play sports and workout at the gym, it all became like a hard struggle for me. So I had to make an appointment for myself at the doctor's to get checked out, to see what was going on with me.

And after the doctors did so many tests on me, they couldn't really figure it out at first. So they started recommending me to other specialist doctors, doctors that went a lot further in their expertise than a regular primary doctor. And once these specialist doctors got through with all the tests they did, they told me I have systemic lupus.

The doctors started to ask me if I had any relatives that have lupus. I said, "Not that I know of." So once I got home, I asked my mom, "Do you have lupus, or does anybody in the family have it?" She said no. So then I called my father to ask him if he had lupus. He said no. Then he said, "Why are you asking?" And I told him, "It's because the doctors said that's what I have, and that's why I'm having these new health issues."

So then he paused for a moment and said, "Okay, so do you know your first cousin, the one who's always laying in the bed when I see her?" I said, "Yes, I know who you're talking about." He said, "Well, she has it. She's been living with lupus for 20 years."

I said, "Wow." And right then and there, I started to feel depressed. I started wondering what was going to happen with me and my future now.

So as you can imagine, I started thinking about how my life was going to change now that I knew I'd be living with lupus. I also started thinking, why me? None of my other brothers or sisters have lupus. Why was I the one chosen for this?

I started to think about all the times I ever told a lie. I started thinking about every time I did something that got me in trouble with my mom, especially all those times I hung out with the same group of friends that kept landing me in trouble in the first place.

Is it because I wouldn't listen when my mom said, "You better stop hanging out with those guys. They are no good role models. They are a bad influence on you. All these guys want to do is smoke cigarettes and go to parties and smoke pot and get into fights. And when they can't handle it all by themselves because they met their match, then they call you to have you finish the fights they started. They're only using you because of your reputation with your boxing skills."

Those words rang in my head over and over again. Was this my punishment? Was this what I deserved for not listening to her warnings?

So I had to make a lot of choices for myself now that I knew I had lupus. And I started by joining a church and cutting those clown guys out of my life. I became mindful about where and when I hang out to enjoy myself.

And then as time went on, I started studying what lupus can do to the body and how to avoid certain situations so that serious medical issues don't get worse. And as I started to get older, I realized that lupus is very unpredictable when it's active. You can do good for two months and then you can do bad for the next two to three months.

When I had bad feelings about why I'm the only one in my family who has lupus, my body would act up, and I'd be in pain. When I thought about doing something that wasn't right (like lying, cheating, hanging out at a club at night, basically getting back with the group of friends Mom told me to stay away from), my health would just be very poor with agonizing pain all over my body. And the pain was so intense it felt like a ten and shot all the way up to a twenty.

But the more I prayed, the more I had good thoughts about everything and everyone, it was like God was sending me signs, telling me to change my lifestyle for the better. And I did just that. And that's when I knew lupus was a blessing, not a curse.

As time went on, I also learned that there are a few different types of lupus.

You have systemic lupus, which is what I have. It's the most common and most serious type.

Then you have cutaneous lupus, which affects the skin, causing rashes, hair loss, and sores.

Then you have drug-induced lupus, which is caused by a reaction to certain prescriptions and medications. It typically disappears after the medications are stopped.

Then you have neonatal lupus, a rare, temporary condition that affects a newborn baby. It occurs when a mother with lupus passes autoantibodies to her child during pregnancy, which can affect the baby's skin, heart, and blood.

Learning all this helped me understand that I wasn't alone in this fight. There were different types, different battles, but we were all warriors in our own way.

So as I started studying more and more about my particular type of lupus, I developed a ritual. I would get out of the shower every morning, look into the mirror, and have a moment with myself. A healing moment where I'd talk to myself and my lupus, trying all types of spiritual healing and prayer therapy.

I started having conversations within myself, saying things like, "Well, it's a blessing to wake up this morning and get my day started with another new journey. And I hope and pray that my lupus will allow my day to run smoothly without any situations that can make me end my day early."

I started feeling a little depressed sometimes. And why I felt like that several times is because you just never know when lupus wants to be very active. So I always have to prepare my mind and body for the worst and the unexpected challenges lupus brings to me while on my journey.

And this is how I started feeling at that moment until I got used to it and decided, well, this is part of how I'll be living my life now. So I had to deal with it and keep my head up and keep it moving. Life goes on until the next journey and chapter of your life.

But I made a promise to myself and to lupus in that mirror. I said, "We are in this together. We will become family and work this journey together and prove to these people we can make it a long journey. We're going to stop all those negative things people are saying about you to me. You and me, lupus, we're a team now."

And from that day forward, that's exactly how I lived my life.

Chapter 2
Getting Through Challenges That Tried to Kill My Faith

I can remember the first time someone gave me negative feedback about lupus like it was yesterday. I was stunned to where I got stuck in my thoughts about what I wanted to do with myself. I really started being stressed out. I started walking around with my head hanging down, never smiling too much anymore, always in a deep depressed mood and deep thought.

People would see me and ask, "Are you alright, Johnny?" And I would say yes, but I was lying. I wasn't alright. I was hurting inside, like my heart was broken and my life was over.

As I sat in my house all alone, I kept replaying all the negative things people were saying to me. Once I told them, "If I don't seem like myself sometimes when I come across you guys, it's because I'm suffering with lupus and it's active right now," they'd be like, "What? What do you mean by active?"

I'd say, "I just found out a couple years back that I was diagnosed with systemic lupus."

And as the word got out to a lot of other individuals I knew, every time I came across one of them, the first thing that came out of their mouth was, "Hey, wassup

Johnny heard you have lupus. I had an aunty who passed away from that. You got to take it easy, Johnny let me know if you need anything, bro."

I used to say, "For one thing, bro, please don't give me any negative conversation about lupus. It's nothing you can catch but something you can inherit from a family member. But I feel if I got it, it's because God wanted me to have it, and I look at it as a blessing from God."

I even remember a time some of the worst words ever spoken to me. They were by the doctor who told me I would die. Can you believe that a doctor told me this?

I will always remember it. It was the worst thing this doctor ever said to me about my lupus diagnosis. This was the moment that almost broke me completely. It came from a doctor in one of the hospitals in Trenton, New Jersey.

He told me to stop asking so many questions. He said, "You do know there's no cure for lupus, just treatment. And just know you are going to die from the lupus. So just keep that in mind, stop being a pest, and let me do my job. I'll give you all the meds for treating it. Thank you."

My heart just fell into my stomach, like someone snatched the life out of me. Almost like all that should be on my mind is, "I am going to die and you just know that, from my lupus." And that definitely had me on edge about telling anyone I had lupus, because then they would treat me just like I have cancer or twenty-four hours to live.

It did not feel good, I tell you. It's a feeling I wish on nobody. Trust me. So, I started shutting down once I started to think about how negativity made me want to hide my lupus.

Since everyone I told about me having lupus always gave me negative feedback, I decided to stop telling anyone. That way I could stop even thinking about having it and still try to live a normal life. Even though I knew I couldn't live completely normal, I always believed that I could, just to keep my faith strong.

I stopped broadcasting it to everyone I met or came in contact with. I kept it to myself, carried the burden alone, because every time I opened up, all I got was more pain, more fear, more reasons to give up. I can remember the turning point at my friend's wedding where a conversation took place that changed my life.

I remember being there and everyone was giving each other compliments about how beautiful the women were in their dresses and how handsome the men were in their tuxedos. It was supposed to be a happy day, a celebration.

And I remember a particular conversation I had with my friend's parents. They were discussing one of their family members who just died from lupus and another family member who wasn't doing well either. In fact, this family member was in the hospital, and they started talking about how every week or every couple of weeks, this family member of theirs just can't get a break from being in and out of the hospital. The doctors that the family member is cared by can't get the lupus under control.

So, once I joined the conversation, I told them, "Maybe I can help give y'all some pointers that work for me."

And they said, "What do you mean, Johnny?"

I said, "Well, I manage myself really well after doing my research and studying other people with it."

Then they said, "What are you saying, Johnny?"

I said, "I am also suffering from lupus, more than twenty years now!"

Everyone, including the ones who weren't in that conversation, was in shock. The whole room seemed to go quiet for a moment. And then my friend's parents were like, "Johnny, I'm so sorry. We had no idea that you have lupus. Oh my God."

I said, "Yes, I just don't go around broadcasting it to everyone I meet or come in contact with."

So, they started asking how I feel, and how I manage it so well to where I hide it so well from other people. And this conversation, this moment of surprise and support instead of negativity, this was different. This was the first time people wanted to learn instead of just telling me horror stories about someone who they know, died from lupus. And this is what inspired my mirror conversations.

I also used to pray to God and say to Him in my prayers, "I know there's got to be a good reason why You put lupus in my life and made it a part of my life journey."

And that's when I started the mirror conversations. I stared into my mirror and talked to myself and the lupus. I needed to see myself, to look myself in the eyes, to have an honest conversation without anyone else's negativity in my thoughts.

I'd tell myself, "I know you're going to give me a very hard life experience to let me know how serious you are." I was saying this to the lupus. "But you will start to ease up on me once you get to know me and I get to know you. And you will see I'm not such a bad person to live with. And you being a blessing from God to be in my life, I will find out the same about you. Because why would God give something to His anointed angel more than they can bear or handle?"

So, the last words in my mirror to lupus were: "We are in this together. We will become family and work this journey together and prove to these people we can make it a long journey, so they can stop the negative things people are saying about you to me."

So, as my journey continues with the battle to find doctors who understood me and my situation, I started to learn what lupus can do to a person's body, I started being introduced to many professionals in that particular field. When I started to have arthritis and pain in all my joints (pain like I never witnessed before in my life), I started getting red rashes from my face throughout my whole body. I started having clots in my blood to the point I had to start taking blood thinners. Sometimes my veins would pop because blood thinners were too strong and I will lose a lot of blood, to where I will have to get blood transfusions. My eyes started getting sensitive to sunlight. I was always tired. As time went on, I started developing new illnesses in multiple parts of my body, so I had to form a family tree of doctors.

And if someone has experienced the same type of suffering in life with some type of treated-only illness that has no cure, when trying to find the right family of doctors, it ain't easy. And yes, from my own experience, I have to break down some of the disturbing situations of what I mean by it ain't easy to find a family of doctors.

Because everyone, including the ones in the professional line of work, don't welcome new patients with open arms, especially people of color who have state insurance and are living on low income. Most of the time, before I got comfortable with new doctors to be treated fairly, it took months, sometimes years, to where they had to get comfortable with me also. To know me and to know I really wanted to be helped and I didn't want no problems either.

A lot of times I was treated unfairly and on the rough side because some of the doctors weren't educated on lupus. They were scared to touch me or even look at my open wounds. They thought they could catch it just by touching me. So, when I was treated like that several times by those doctors, most of the times back-to-back, I just kept giving up. I didn't want to even deal with no more doctors.

I tried to develop my own home remedies to treat myself by reading lots of books on other people's testimonials and looking at websites, studying all types of herbs and spices to treat different organs in my body. And so on and so on. I still was searching for the right doctors on my journey. And yes, oh boy, oh boy, there were plenty of moments I almost gave up as well.

Don't think for one moment I didn't think about giving up. I always thought about giving up for so long. It was a very big challenging situation for me to break away from. But it just seems the more I prayed to be strong, the more I prayed to God to help me fight harder than I ever did in my life. And every hour, every day, every week, it took years for me to overcome all the weak moments.

I'd set back and think about how my life used to be before lupus came into my life. I broke down many times for years.

But then I started always thinking of the people in my life, the ones who surrounded me with love. I thought about the people who cared about my situation more than me. I thought about people who were fighting harder than me for my well-being. And that's what pulled me back every single time.

And I said to myself, "I can't let their hard work go to waste. I can't let people who love me be a waste of their time. All the praying they did for me and running around to help with some of my important needs and living situations. No, no, no! I had to get mad at myself and pull it together and get back on the wagon and get back to reality finding God through all of this first.

I tell you, I really ended up getting a really good, close relationship with God from dealing with lupus. That's why I will always be thankful for lupus most of the time. I never thought in a million years that having a relationship with God could feel so good, inside and out.

I used to always read the scriptures in my Bible, like twice a day, to help with my healing also. Scriptures like:

Exodus 15:26: "I am the Lord, who heals you."

Psalm 103:3: "Who forgives all your sins and heals all your diseases."

Isaiah 53:5: "By His wounds we are healed."

Yes, those scriptures most of the time got me through the hard moments.

They were my lifeline when I felt like I was drowning in reality. I had to start learning how to work with lupus. And because of how I live my life now with lupus, that's how I decided to always have conversations with lupus, to always be aware of what it brings to me in my life. And I also at that time decided that me and the lupus will have to work together, because I am not going out without a fight!

It took years, I'm not going to lie. Years of fighting, years of breaking down, years of building myself back up. But slowly, I started to understand that lupus wasn't my enemy. It was my teacher, my wake-up call, my guardian angel in disguise.

So, I started sharing my home remedies with family and friends at weddings. I would share what I personally do for myself. And I want to share them with you too:

You have to believe you will be alright. You have to have strong faith in yourself and God, that He wouldn't put lupus in your life if He knew you couldn't handle it.

You have to do your own studies on lupus, because even though the doctors are professionals in their field, they themselves are still studying different symptoms that come from lupus.

You yourself must never sit back and dwell on your life, feeling sorry for yourself or letting yourself get in a depressed mood. Try changing your diet and the way you eat and sleep. Know how many hours of sleep you should get on a regular basis. Stay out of high-temperature sunlight.

Try your best not to let no one steal your joy or knock down your high spirits. Meditate. Have spiritual conversations with yourself and God in the mirror or in your mind while reading a Bible or reading someone else's success stories.

You must get that mindset of keeping your life going on, no matter what people may say that's negative or what you might think of what's to come to you that can be negative. You want to make that your biggest battle with lupus: avoiding any and everything that can be negativity to your mind, body, and spiritual soul.

And this is what I would tell someone who has just been diagnosed with lupus.

Whenever I hear of someone just getting to know lupus in their life, I tell them to just accept it and look at it as a blessing from God. I did after knowing it, and how it definitely changed my life for the best, in my beliefs.

But when I hear someone not having good thoughts about lupus when they discover they have it, I will tell them this:

Listen, I know you're scared. I know people are telling you horror stories. I know that doctor might have made you feel like your life is over. But let me tell you something: you are stronger than you think. God doesn't make mistakes. If He gave you lupus, He also gave you the strength to handle it.

Keep up with your doctors, your rheumatologist, your kidney specialists, and your primary doctors. These doctors, after a while, become your family, your friends, and a guardian angel in so many ways.

At the same time, do your own research and studying every chance you get. It's a must, especially if you still want to cope with some of the normal lifestyle that you lived at a time in your life.

And always keep the number one rule in your life journey: Stay away from negative news on TV, from the people you know and don't know. Don't watch depressed movies or TV shows that talk about someone who just died or someone who is suffering and just gave up without a fight. Stay focused on all positive things to keep your mindset at ease and full of happy thoughts.

You've got this. And if you ever feel like giving up, remember: there's a Master Barber Chef Doctor named Johnny who's been living with lupus for over twenty years, and he's not just surviving, he's thriving. And if I can do it, so can you.

Chapter 3
Cooking: The Blessing in My Life

Making changes to what I eat and how I eat, every meal had to become a special treat to meet my needs. That's what my lupus was telling me. When I started eating anything and everything that wasn't right for my body and mind, my lupus and I would be fussing with each other.

You know what I'm talking about, people? If you're not feeling well for some particular reason, you find yourself cursing, saying stuff like, "Damn, what's going on? Shhhhh, I was feeling good all the other days. Where did this sickness come from?"

Well, I tell you, like the old saying goes; you are what you eat. You best believe that. So let me tell you about my favorite meal.

I can remember a meal that I loved to make on a Friday. This was back before lupus changed everything about how I ate, how I lived, and how I thought about food.

I used to make baked barbecue beef ribs, smothered in onions, drowning in mustard and barbecue sauce, with a side of Spanish yellow rice and homemade butter biscuits. And I'd make myself a large vanilla and banana milkshake.

That was my favorite meal to have on a Friday night when watching my favorite old black and white classic American movie. Yes, I love to watch old classic gangster and mystery movies, especially horror movies. They remind me of when my mom used to have all the family together eating our favorite foods and snacks.

That meal, that ritual, that Friday night feeling of being full and satisfied and entertained, that was my life before lupus made me change everything, especially the way I look at rich foods. I knew it all would come to an end some day. I knew I would have to change the way I eat and think now. I just knew I had to start some where and so I started cooking with the purpose to change things for the better.

A lot of things started to change as I started cooking with a purpose. I became much happier than ever; smiling a lot more, with more willpower to go on living and enjoying life like any other individual who was full of life in so many ways.

I had to become my own nutritionist, studying every medication and substituting it for a fruit or vegetable that met some of the same needs and produced some of the same ingredients as some of the medications I was taking.

Like I said before, I started my own home remedies. Now, I'm not telling you to go and run with what I'm telling you, but I'm just sharing what worked for me at that time. Yes, I used my own remedies to hold me down until I found a doctor I could feel comfortable with, someone who had lots of education on my lupus because this was my new life.

I also started watching real-life experiences and documentaries of people who survived their childhood struggles and lived to tell their stories. And matter of fact, that is one of my therapy sessions: watching inspirational gospel shows and movies. No more gangster films. No more violence and negativity filling my mind while I eat. Now it's inspiration, it's survival stories, it's people who overcame.

I'll make my favorite food, putting in colorful fruits and vegetables that bring me joy. I'll top it off with salmon smothered in garlic butter and herbs with leafy spinach, or some chicken liver and onions with homemade mushroom gravy, with some whole wheat toast and a small, tossed salad; the spring mix type with blueberries, raspberries, strawberries, and diced up watermelon.

I can't wait to go to town on it every time. It tastes so good, like if it was my first time making this dish. And I always went to sleep not feeling bloated or full, but just right. And nothing on my mind but how good that food I just ate was. And I always managed to get a good night's sleep.

After discovering what foods triggered my lupus, I started to realize, every time I made a certain dish, it would have a different reaction on my health.

When I made food like fish, chicken, and liver with mixed vegetables, I felt so alive and full of energy. I could get up in the morning ready to take on the day. I could walk without my joints screaming at me. I could think clearly without brain fog clouding everything.

But when I cooked food like thick beef steaks, hefty beef burgers and pork chops with baked potato or fried French fries or white rice and beans, I felt sluggish and down in a depressed mood and just wanting to sleep. My body would ache. My head would hurt. My joints would swell up. It was like my lupus was punishing me for eating that way.

And that's how I started realizing what made my lupus want to be active. So I had to make a choice on how I wanted to feel from now on, and I started eating healthy. I had to start becoming my own nutritionist.

I spent most of my time in fruit and vegetable markets, shopping for varieties of fruits and vegetables. I started to discover so many fruits and vegetables that I had never seen before or heard of.

And after a while, it started being fun for me and became part of my daily routine exercises, almost like my private therapy session. This is how I always started my day in the morning hours.

And I tell you, it wasn't easy trying to get a healthy program going on with yourself. It took a lot of discipline, and most of all, money that you have on you at that time for shopping for healthy foods.

And once you kind of get your program of healthy eating going on, you will definitely start to enjoy it and

your life. And you will always tell yourself, "I can't believe I've been missing out on all these good-tasting,
wonderful foods that are good for the body and mind.
And all this time I thought it was hamburgers and fries
or Philly cheesesteaks and fried onion rings." That's a
joke.

I started making and inventing all types of fruit salads
and vegetable salads, even assorted peanut salads, especially if you like crunchiness. So I started eating certain fruits and vegetables for my eyes and hair and skin
and for the inflammation that was making my joints
pain like crazy.

I tried concentrating on what part of my muscles in my
body gave me the most problems. That's one of the
ways I would do my shopping for fruits and vegetables.
If my joints were hurting bad that week, I'd look up
what foods fight inflammation. If my eyes were sensitive to light, I'd research what vitamins help with eye
health. If my skin was breaking out in rashes, I'd find
out what foods promote skin healing.

It's definitely a big process trying to keep your new lifestyle in order, because that's what it becomes after a
while for yourself: a whole new life to adjust to and
maintain to your best ability.

A typical day of eating on the regular is like an adven-
ture! And I say this because of the fact that I can't wait
until I try out new fruits and vegetables that I discovered on the internet.

I do research on all new fruits and vegetables I add to my diet. I see the reasons people eat it more than three to four times a week, and I find out that it could control your blood pressure or inflammation, and also be a good healthy benefit for your heart and other organs.

I do research so much for my body parts that give me the problems and pain. It's like I really had to become my own home doctor. It is so fun to explore different recipes for the food you eat. I like to discover what island, what country this fruit or vegetable is from, why it is so popular, and why people eat certain seafood dishes all the time instead of meats.

This is how I live my life now, and this is how I discovered the fruits and vegetables that can help keep down my inflammation. This is another reason why I like the supermarket therapy because it is where my healing begins every morning.

I love going to the markets just to be around different fruits and vegetables because of their colors and the atmosphere itself. To be surrounded by all your favorite fruits and vegetables and people that are doing the same thing you do, it is an important part of my physical therapy.

I do this mostly every day, even if it's only buying a bag of grapes. The smell of fresh flowers and food that some supermarkets will have, a place where they cook food to sell to the customers. And to walk around the supermarket and look at all the different tossed salads and baked cakes and the sales they will have with the food you like to buy.

It became my morning routine, my meditation, my way of starting the day right. Some people go to the gym. Some people go for a jog. I go to the fruit market to the produce section and let the colors and smell of tropical citrus fruits and possibilities of healing me before I even get home.

The temptation still stands face to face with me in those supermarkets.

I see a lot of food that I used to eat when I was younger, and I get so tempted to cheat a little bit. But I can't. I've come a long way with being disciplined with myself and foods.

I used to love a lot of pork and beef, and I mean the down South type of food, the Southern styles: cornbread, baked mac and cheese, pork chops and gravy, pig's feet and chitterlings, hog, ham, turkey necks.

I really didn't want to give up that rich type of eating. But I had to make a choice. Did I want to feel good inside or corrupted inside? I went with the good inside because it just felt better to feel that way.

And let me tell you, standing in that supermarket, looking at those fried chicken wings, and smelling that cornbread from the bakery section, seeing that mac and cheese in the deli, it takes everything in me not to put it in my cart. But then I remember how I felt after eating that way. I remember the pain. I remember the sluggishness. I remember lupus winning. And I put it back and walk to the produce section where healing lives and the feeling of goodness begins.

To be able to live with that healthy diet is very expensive! That's the truth. Nobody wants to have to keep buying fresh salmon, organic berries, spring mix salads, whole wheat bread and almond nuts.

I have a way to keep up with my healthy eating by shopping for deals. I try breaking down a lot of spending habits that's not worth spending money on. And I don't always have to eat three times a day, like breakfast, lunch, and dinner.

I'll just eat a light breakfast or a light dinner and an okay lunch. Or just eat an okay breakfast, skip lunch, and then just have dinner. That way I can keep up with the healthy food that I now do eat. Quality over quantity, that became my motto. I tell you

Who said keeping up with a healthy lifestyle was easy? The hardest part of this is when your body goes through withdrawals. It's probably one of the hardest things to do in life, next to trying to have a successful future, a long-term relationship, or having a healthy marriage without marriage counseling.

If something you're doing in life doesn't make you happy or looks like it isn't worth the hard work, you will end up giving up. And I believe that a lot of people's problems chang their lifestyle for the better. They come out being the best version of themselves

Me, myself, just taking things in life for granted, it just wasn't working for me. I found myself year after year going in a circle of the same routine, just different times and days and different people.

I can remember when I first started to eat on a diet and started eating healthy foods, my body was going through a depressed mood because it was craving for that fast food, that junk food type. I really thought I wasn't going to be able to handle it or even do it.

My body was literally going through withdrawal like I was coming off drugs. I'd wake up at night craving a cheeseburger. I'd drive past McDonald's and almost pull in. I'd smell some Caribbean food and almost lost my mind. Yes, it was that serious.

But I did it. I pushed through it. And after a few weeks, the cravings got easier. After a few months, I didn't even want that food anymore. My body had adjusted to the new normal, the new life that was about to begin.

My advice for others who are trying to do what I am doing is to start slow and build discipline. It's just as simple as that.

I will tell anyone who's about to change their diet to a healthy diet to start slow and train themselves to be disciplined. Try to think of eating healthy as a must, because if you don't, you won't be as successful in the future. You will not feel your best. You will not look your best or live your best life.

It is overwhelming, but you have to stick with it and just do it. Don't try to change everything overnight. Start with one meal. Start with breakfast. Once you get that down, move to lunch. Then dinner. Then snacks.

Don't beat yourself up if you cheat once in a while. Just get back on track the next meal. Progress, not perfection. That's what matters. You taking the first step, taking time for yourself, setting boundaries and making progress is what is going to help you heal yourself.

Sometimes I would tell myself, "I'm tired of repeating the same routine year after year, not feeling good, always depressed and stressed out of my mind. Something's got to give."

So I really had to take a stand and take some time away from everyone and everything to get a clearer vision of my life. I mean, no more phone calls from people who are always trying to dump their problems on me or get me involved in their problems.

And this is one of the other reasons all these changes came about. I realized that stress was triggering my lupus just as much as bad food was. I had to protect my peace. I had to protect my energy. I had to say no to people, situations, and yes to myself, even food that wasn't serving me a purpose. I was just leaving it alone.

That meant turning off my phone sometimes. That meant not answering every call. That meant saying, "I can't help you with that right now, I'm working on myself." And you know what? Some people understood. Some people didn't. But the ones who really loved me supported my boundaries always understood where I was coming from.

It transformed me. Looking back now, I can't believe the difference. Before I changed my diet, I was in pain every single day. I was taking too much over the medication. I was exhausted all the time. I was depressed. I was giving up.

After I changed my diet, the inflammation went down. The pain decreased. I had energy again. I could think clearly. I could smile genuinely. I could see a future.

It wasn't overnight. It took months to see real change. But it happened. And it was worth every temptation I resisted, every dollar I spent on fresh produce, every morning I woke up and went to that market instead of that drive-through.

Food became my medicine. Cooking became my therapy. The kitchen became my laboratory where I experimented with healing. And slowly but surely, I became the Master Barber Chef Doctor not just in title, but in practice. I was doctoring myself back to health, one meal at a time. Thank God for his blessings and will power.

Chapter 4
Recreating Myself After Lupus Changed My Work Life

So now you know I had to change the way I eat because of lupus. But I also had to change the way I received my income. I still had to take care of myself and still pay bills.

I wasn't able to work a nine-to-five anymore once the lupus started being very active on a regular basis. Even though I was eating the right food, that wasn't enough!

I still had to learn how to control the lupus, or get it under control in doctor's terms. I had to try to learn how to put the lupus to sleep if I wanted to get a steady flow going on with what I was working on during the travels of my journey.

Before I get into how I recreated myself, let me tell you about the job I lost that started this whole journey of reinvention.

My nine-to-five job was at a restaurant where I worked from being a teenager until I became a young adult. I loved that job. Man, I really loved it. Being in the kitchen, cooking for people, seeing their faces light up when they tasted the food I made, that was everything to me. It was my passion, my purpose, working with food every single day. I thought I'd work there forever. I thought I'd be one of those old cooks who retires after 40 years of service.

But then I had to leave because of the varicose veins in my legs. They made my legs swell up terribly and put me in a lot of pain. The standing, the constant moving around the hot kitchen, the long shifts - my body just couldn't take it anymore. So I had to quit my job because of it.

My boss didn't understand anything about varicose veins. He was not educated on how it worked, how serious it could get, and what it did to your body. All he kept telling me was, "If you don't fix the problems with your health and get yourself in shape, I need someone who can work full-time and part-time, six days a week. I need somebody reliable."

I kept telling him, "Listen, I've been to four different doctors, and they all told me the same thing. I can't be on my feet for a long period of time. I have to take it easy until they can get my blood circulation under control. This is serious."

But he didn't want to hear it. So he told me he would have to take away most of my days. And he did. He only gave me one day a week to work. Just one day. After all the years I put in at that restaurant, after all the meals I cooked, after all the customers I satisfied, after all the times I came in early and stayed late, I was down to one single day a week.

That hurt. That hurt a lot.

On that particular day I went to work. I remember it was on a Saturday morning. I was standing in the kitchen of the restaurant prepping food to cook, getting everything ready for the lunch rush, and something felt weird at the bottom of my legs. Like a strange pressure, a warmth that wasn't normal.

I looked down to see what was wrong, and I saw a pile of blood gushing from my left leg. Just pouring out. Come to find out, my vein had popped from me standing too long!

The kitchen erupted. People screaming, someone calling 911, my coworkers trying to help me sit down. Blood everywhere on the floor, on my shoes, pooling around me. It looked like a crime scene.

They had to call the ambulance and rush me to the emergency room. The paramedics tried to apply pressure to the vein that had popped, but they couldn't stop the blood from coming out because I was on blood thinners for the blood clots in my legs. And the small hole where the vein was, was kind of big. It was big enough to where it needed five small stitches in order for them to stop the bleeding.

After they stopped the bleeding, they discovered I'd lost a lot of blood to where I needed a blood transfusion! I ended up staying four days in the hospital before being discharged. Four days of lying there thinking about my life, about my future, about what in the world I was going to do now.

After I got home, I called my boss and told him I would not be returning to work. I was done. I couldn't risk that happening again.

And you know what he said? He told me, "Yes, please don't come back because I can't be taking chances with you. What happened scared the customers. That's bad for business."

That was it. No "I hope you're okay." No "Thank you for your years of service." Just "Don't come back."

That was a scary moment. Many customers were asking a lot of questions about what happened, about all
the blood, about the ambulance coming. Some of them
saw it happen. It was traumatic for everyone there.

But you know what? It was also a wake-up call.

I started thinking about what happened at my job and
decided I didn't want no more of that type of situation.
So I'd better learn what was going on with my health
issues in my legs. What was my body trying to tell me?
What were the limits I needed to respect?

And yes, once I started to learn all what lupus can do, I
found out I would not be able to work a regular job, especially one that would cause me to do any long standing and walking and going up and down a lot of stairs.

So once I found out it would be tough knowing I can't
work the jobs I love, like restaurants, because of my
love of cooking, it made me feel my life was definitely
going to be different and depressing for me. And just to
know I wouldn't be able to do a lot of activities I like,
especially with my legs' condition, it was like, "Man,
what type of life will I be living now? Who am I if I'm
not a cook? What am I supposed to do with myself as
time goes on?

The dark days came and went and all I wanted to do
was sleep but I had to go to physical therapy because
the lupus would have my whole body in a lot of pain.
I'm talking about pain that makes you not want to
move, pain that makes you not want to get out of bed,
pain that makes you wonder if it's even worth it to keep
fighting.

All I wanted to do was lay in bed, take my medications, and sleep. Sleep through the pain. Sleep through the depression. Sleep through the questions about my future. Until I realized I was just sleeping my life away.

So I used to force myself to get up and fight my way back into the world of civilization and start coping with life. I'd set an alarm. I'd count to three. I'd throw the covers off before I could talk myself out of it. Because if I didn't, I could see myself really suffering at its worst.

The stories people told me about their loved ones and what they went through because they just gave up on themselves. I just couldn't do it. I couldn't become another sad story people told at weddings. My mind was too determined to not let lupus run my life. So I started praying very hard to God and I believe those prayers gave me the strength to keep fighting.

I prayed every day. Every single day. Even on the days I didn't feel like it, I prayed. Every day I saw myself getting stronger. The more I talked to God spiritually while praying, I started getting a much clearer picture of how I wanted to see my life getting back on track, doing normal things people do, like wanting more out of life, wanting to actually live life instead of just surviving it.

And going back to school was my first step forward. I started to look into going back, and I received my high school diploma online. That was my first victory. My first real achievement after everything fell apart. After losing my restaurant job, after that vein popping in the kitchen, after all those dark days in bed thinking my life was over, I got my high school diploma.

I proved to myself I could still learn. I could still grow. I could still achieve something. My body might be broken, but my mind was still sharp and strong. So I decided to go to barber school.

I started going to NYC American Barbers in Manhattan and worked toward receiving my Master Barber License. This was it. This was going to be my new career. I could sit while I worked. No more standing for eight hours. No more swollen legs. No more risk of veins popping.

And just when I thought I knew it all going to that barber school, let me tell you, it's a lot more than you think there is to know. I thought barbering was just cutting hair. I was wrong.

I had to first learn how to clean and properly sanitize my barbershop tools. I had to learn how to recognize certain diseases in someone's hair, like lice and other diseases hair would carry. I had to know when to refuse service to protect myself and other clients.

I had to learn people's body language, to see if this person would be an easy haircut or a difficult one to cut and groom. You can tell a lot about a client before they even sit in your chair. Are they fidgety? Are they looking at their phone the whole time? Are they making eye contact? All of that tells you what kind of experience you're about to have.

I had to study different types of hairstyle languages and slang talk, and the way they would use the popular slang talk in different parts of a state or country. And when I say slang talk, I mean words like: someone will ask for a "mid fade," someone else will probably just say, "Little off the sides and keep it low," and someone else might say, "Clean me up," and they all mean something slightly different. You have to learn to speak the language of hair.

The more I learned from the barbering school I attended, it was definitely another new type of learning experience for me, especially when you have to deal with so many different styles of people, from different nationalities and countries and religions. Different hair textures. Different expectations. Different cultural standards of what looks good.

It was tough, but I did it. I passed the Master Barber exams and achieved my Master Barber License. I held that certificate in my hands and felt like I had my life back. I had a future again I couldn't wait to get my first barbering.

And when I did get my first job at a barbershop, I was so excited to actually be working there professionally. This was it. I found it. The perfect job for someone with lupus. I could sit while I worked. No more standing on my legs for hours. No more swelling. No more pain. I could cut hair, make people look good, make money, and take care of my health all at the same time.

I thought I finally figured it out. I thought I finally found my solution.

And then COVID came around. I had to leave the barbershop because they all were being closed down because of COVID. Just like that, the world shut down. And my perfect solution disappeared overnight so I had to come up with another solution.

So I came up with an idea to keep my income coming. I started to make house calls and did haircuts outside the client's house. If people couldn't come to the barbershop, I'd bring the barbershop to them. I started going to people's houses to cut their hair and to their place of work. I put my clippers in a bag, loaded up my car, and became a mobile barber. It wasn't an easy thing to deal with, because of no rules outside of a barbershop, most people will do what people do what they want, and that is not stay still, answering the phone, and worst of all, smoking a cigarette while getting a haircut.

And it wasn't easy during the time I was cutting people's hair at their houses. It would be in the front yard or backyard or garage, and everyone had a cigarette in their mouth. So I'm cutting hair with one eye open because I was in the middle of ten to fifteen people smoking at the same time. The smoke burning my eyes, making me cough, going into my lungs.

I couldn't tell them to put the cigarettes out because I didn't want to lose their business. So I had to put up with a lot also, just to make ends meet.

But you know what? I have a Master Barber License. I went to school for this. I passed exams for this. And here I am cutting hair in somebody's backyard while they blow cigarette smoke in my face like I'm nothing. Like my health doesn't matter. Like my professionalism doesn't deserve respect.

I felt so disrespected to where I said, "I'll leave this alone for a while until I can find a better class of people who I can do business with. I don't have to put up with this nonsense.

When the barbershop business was slowing down because people were getting scared to get a haircut because they thought they could catch COVID, now I had to come up with another plan. Again. Always another plan. Always adapting. Always pivoting.

So I went into getting my taxi registration, and I got a job driving a taxi. Maybe thinking that was the answer. Maybe this was finally it. Sitting down all day, driving people around, making money without standing on my legs. No hot kitchens. No cigarette smoke. Just driving.

And I remember my first ride was fun and exciting. I felt like, "This is it! I can do this. No standing, no walking. I think I'll be okay. This might actually work."

But then I started to see a lot of unexpected problems come with this type of job also. So as I started to work more and more with the taxi services, I ran into lots of people who you would never think would try to scam you. People who look normal, people who dress nice, people who smile and make conversation. And then try to steal from you.

I can remember an older lady was picking up her son from school, and he was about five or six years old. Nice-looking woman. Well-dressed. Looked like a good mother. The woman flagged me down to stop and use my taxi services. She had me take her home, and then the unexpected happened.

She pretended to go in her purse to get the taxi fare, and then opened the door and jumped out, leaving her kid behind, telling him, "Just come on, run, run! Hurry!"

And not only was I in shock, but the kid was also in shock. That's why he froze up, like, "Mommy, what are you doing? What is going on? What's happening with you?"

I couldn't believe it. A mother using her own child as a distraction to steal a taxi ride. What kind of person does that? What kind of mother teaches her child to run from honest people trying to make a living?

Then there was a time when another woman used my taxi services. She waited until I got her to her designated area, and when she gave me the taxi fare, she balled up the money and shoved it in my hand and rushed to get out of my taxi.

And when I opened the money, I found it was only three dollars! The fare was seven dollars.

I jumped out of my taxi and told the woman, "You're supposed to pay me seven dollars. You're four dollars short."

She claimed to not know any English. Started shaking her head, saying things I couldn't understand, pretending she had no idea what I was talking about.

So I said, "Okay." I didn't want to argue. I didn't want to make a scene. I took a loss of a few dollars and drove away. What else could I do?

But you know what? God has a sense of humor.

I ended up seeing her a couple days later, and it was snowing so hard and the ground was covered with five feet of snow. The wind was blowing. The roads were barely drivable. And there she was on the corner, flagging me down.

And guess what? This time she spoke very clearly in English. Perfect English. "Taxi! Taxi! Please, I need a ride! It's so cold!"

But this time I rolled down my window and said, "No, sorry, I don't speak any English," and I pulled off. Let someone else deal with her. Let her stand in five feet of snow. She wanted to play games with me, now she could stand out in a blizzard.

I watched her in my rearview mirror, standing there looking confused, and I smiled. Sometimes karma comes quick. After a while I couldn't just do that anymore so I started cooking weekend dinners and selling them for a low price just to get people to buy the food. I was using every skill I had. Cooking. Cutting hair. Driving. Whatever it took to pay the bills and keep my head above water.

And as you know, a lot of side hustles don't last long. The taxi job had too many scammers and not enough money after gas and maintenance. The house call haircuts had too many disrespectful clients. The weekend dinners were too inconsistent; some weekends I'd sell out, other weekends barely anyone would buy.

So I just started hanging within the NYC five boroughs. I started doing freelancing where I would visit friends I knew who had their own barbershop, and I'd hang out and do a little haircutting. Not a full schedule, just helping out, making some money, keeping my skills sharp.

And I would also cook a nice food spread at home and bring it with me to the barbershop by request only, because everyone knows there's nothing like getting something to eat after getting cleaned up with a haircut. Fresh cut, fresh meal. That's how you feel like a new man.

That's when I started to see it. The connection between what I do. The way cooking and barbering actually complement each other. The way both are about making people feel good about themselves. So I started putting two to three dreams together in one platform, which is one let me do a little modeling since that was my first ever real spotlight gig at a teenager to get discovered, two I work in so many restaurants I always thought it will be nice to have my own in sometime in life, so after a while from finding out my father comes from a family tree of barbers, I figure well let me go to barber school get my license, because I did do this in my life at a time ,and was good at it especially when my mind was clear and heart was happy.

Another dream was to have my own barbershop restaurant.

That is one of my passions; to someday own my own barbershop slash restaurant, where you can come get a haircut and walk to the next side to get something to eat. Or while you're waiting to get your haircut, spend time in the restaurant side eating a good meal.

Picture it: You walk in, you check in for your haircut, and while you're waiting, you order from the menu. Maybe some salmon or some organic chicken breast covered with leafy spinach. Or maybe some chicken with mixed vegetables. Maybe a fruit salad with berries and watermelon. Something healthy. Something that makes you feel good inside while you're getting cleaned up outside.

Then your name gets called, you get your haircut, you look in the mirror and see a new you. And on your way out, you can grab your food to go or sit and eat it right there. Or maybe you eat first, then get your haircut. Either way it will works.

That's my vision. That's my goal. A place where I can use both of my skills without having to choose, without having to pivot, without having to give one up for the other. The Master Barber Chef Doctor, slash model, finally living up to the full name. Finally bringing everything together in one place. Because I always thought and wanted to become my own boss.

So I started thinking on being-my-own-boss levels from the time I started doing my own research on my lupus. And the more I educated myself on it, I just knew it wasn't going to be the same, me trying to be employed in someone else's place of business.

I couldn't work for people who didn't understand lupus. I couldn't work for people who cut my hours when I got sick. I couldn't work for people who told me not to come back after my vein popped in their kitchen. I couldn't work for people who expected me to stand for eight hours when my body couldn't handle it. I couldn't work for people who saw me as disposable, as replaceable, as just another employee who could be let go without a second thought.

I had to be my own boss. I had to control my own schedule. I had to decide when I worked and when I rested. I had to create a life that worked around my lupus, not try to force my lupus to work around someone else's business demands.

That's not hustle culture. That's not some motivational speaker telling you to "be your own boss" because it sounds good. That's survival. That's adaptation. That's necessity. But that's the journey of reinventing myself and that is what this chapter is really about. It's not just about losing jobs and finding new ones. It's about completely reinventing yourself when your body tells you that you can't live the life you planned. It's about getting knocked down and getting back up, over and over and over again, until you finally figure out a way to stay standing.

Let me show you the pattern:

Restaurant cook → Vein popped, forced to leave

Dark days in bed → Forced myself to get up and pray

Got high school diploma online → First victory after trauma

Went to barbering school → New skill, new hope, new future

Got barbershop job → Perfect solution for lupus (sitting job)

COVID shut everything down → Back to square one

House call haircuts → Disrespectful clients smoking in my face

Taxi driver → Scammers, thieves, people using kids to steal

Weekend dinner sales → Inconsistent, unreliable income

Freelance barber/chef → Finally finding some balance

Dream of barbershop/restaurant → Vision for the future

Every time I thought I found the answer, something happened. But I kept adapting. I kept changing. I kept fighting. I kept praying. I kept believing God had a plan even when I couldn't see it.

Because that's what you do when you have lupus and bills to pay. You don't give up. You reinvent. You hustle. You pray. You find another way. And then when that way gets blocked, you find another way. And another. And another.

Through all of that; the blood, the scams, the smoke, the setbacks, the disappointments, the rejections, I kept my faith. I prayed every day. I talked to God. I got stronger. I got my diploma. I got my license. I kept my dream alive.

And I'm still here. Still standing. Still fighting. Still the Master Barber Chef Doctor.

Still Johnny.

Chapter 5
Pulling All My Strength to Keep My Journey Moving

A lot of times when trying to stay focused on my journey into completing the mission of reaching my goals, I used to get sidetracked and thrown off. I would be feeling stuck in the moment wondering if it's worth the pain and suffering.

The reason why I'm saying this is because during the whole time my body is aching from open sores on my ankles. My legs are swollen and toes are numb and aching, and I just didn't want to be feeling more pain. The thought of getting out of bed to clean the open wounds and wrap them up with the gauze, that process alone takes up to an hour or an hour and a half. My stomach was always hurting me. I had headaches. My finger joints were in pain because of arthritis. It was just so hard to keep putting up with all of that just to get my day going.

After a while dealing with the varicose veins in my legs, them being swollen and still not under control, I was still in the learning process of getting the swelling to reduce. So one day I tried to get out of bed and do some stretching for my legs, thinking that it might help me. But it was really hard because of the simple fact that my legs were too sore and I was in so much pain. My ankles, my calves, my toes were all numb. Everything throughout my whole body was stiff, and it was like arthritis throughout all of my body parts.

So for a while, it always took me fifteen to twenty minutes to get out of bed completely. Just to sit up. Just to swing my legs over the side. Just to touch my feet to the floor.

I had to sit myself up by pulling on my bed rail. Then I'd grab the closest chair to me and use it as a support item because I had no walking cane at that time. I would use the chair and part of the bed rail to walk very slowly until I could get into the kitchen and grab onto another chair. And I would use my two chairs to walk myself to the bathroom, holding myself up by leaning on the wall to get around the house and get what I needed for myself. Like when it was time for a drink of water, or fixing myself something to eat, or taking my medications.

Using two chairs like a makeshift walker. That's where I was at. That's what lupus had reduced me to.

As I would clean the open wounds on my legs, I just couldn't believe I actually was going through this type of situation and suffering! I didn't think of something like this in a million years. Every time when it was time to change the wrappings on my wounds, I'd cry. Shaking my head, hanging down, saying, "This can't be real. What is going on? Did someone put a curse on me or wish my life will be like this, to make me suffer? So I can see and feel what suffering is all about?"

So it always took me about 40 to 45 minutes just to clean up my wounds and wrap them up. And another 30 to 40 minutes to put on the surgical socks over the wrapping. The simple fact is because my legs would still be swelling, and with the gauzes and wrappings, it made the width bigger. So I had to struggle pulling them up and over, all the way up to my knees. And it would hurt really, really badly, to the point where I had to lay down for another 30 minutes or more until my legs could adjust to the wrapping and the surgical socks.

Let me break down that process for you:

First, I had to unwrap the old bandages. That alone was painful because the gauze would stick to the open sores, and pulling it off felt like ripping my skin.

Second, I had to clean each wound with saline solution or whatever the doctor prescribed. Touching open sores, cleaning out any drainage, making sure nothing was infected. That's 20 minutes right there.

Third, I had to apply the ointment or medication the doctor prescribed. Gently, carefully, trying not to cause more pain.

Fourth, I had to wrap each leg with fresh gauze, making sure it was tight enough to compress but not so tight it cut off circulation.

Fifth, I had to pull those surgical compression socks over the wrapped legs. And let me tell you, those socks are TIGHT. When your legs are already swollen and wrapped in gauze, getting those socks on feels impossible. I'd pull and tug and struggle, and the pain would shoot through my legs so bad I'd have to stop and breathe.

The whole process? An hour and a half. Sometimes two hours if I had to rest in between because the pain was too much.

And I had to do this every single day. Every. Single. Day.

Because of this I couldn't wear any shoes. I mostly wore a pair of slippers. All summer, all winter. All around my hometown to my doctor appointments and back and forth to the supermarket. I even went as far as to NYC, riding the trains, up and down the subways, all the way to Brooklyn to my girlfriend's grandmother and father's house, when it was below 20 degrees!

I did it because I wanted to make sure she got there safely when she used to go visit her family and friends. People would stare at me like I was losing my mind because I was up and around all through NYC's five boroughs during the coldest time of the year, wearing slippers.

Slippers. In below 20-degree weather. In the middle of winter. On the subway. Walking through Brooklyn.

Sometimes I'd look down at myself during that time, at my fingers, and I would be like, "Wow, my fingers are turning blue." My lips turned blue. My face turned reddish blue. That's how cold it was. And I was just hacking it out as much as I could. And I did this routine for about two years, so I was almost getting immune to it. But not quite. The cold still hurt. The pain was still there. But I did it anyway because she needed me and I needed her.

At times I would just lay in bed with my eyes open, staring at the wall, at the ceiling. And after a while, I'd close my eyes and start praying to God for strength. That's what seems to help me most of the times.

And after a while, while praying, I start to get a warmish feeling traveling throughout my whole body. Like
my body is being renewed. Or like the Spirit of God is
inside of me, helping me get up and out of the bed, telling me, "If we stick together, we can do this. Let's go."

Every day I prayed before leaving my house and starting my mission for the day. And when I prayed, it felt
like God was sending a strong warmish feeling, but also
a strong vibration type of feeling. Almost like a magical
whole new spirit just jumped into my body and gave me
strength all throughout my body. Like I never felt any
pain nor arthritis in any parts of my body.

It's hard to describe unless you've felt it yourself. But
it's like this: you're lying there in pain, everything
hurts, you don't want to move. And then you close your
eyes and start talking to God. And slowly, you feel this
warmth starting in your chest and spreading out. Not
like heat from a blanket. Not like warmth from coffee.
But like an internal warmth, like your blood is warming
up from the inside. And with that warmth comes this
vibration, this energy, this strength.

And suddenly, you can move. The pain is still there, but
you can push through it. Your legs still hurt, but you
can stand. Your joints still ache, but you can walk.

That's the power of God. That's one of the true blessings God would show me in so many ways. He's in control, no matter what you're going through. This was one
part of my morning routine.

After that I would get up and start making my black
coffee to help warm up my joints and get my orange
juice to take my medications. And I make myself a vitamin booster snack, which will be 12 grain bread, one

slice, spread peanut butter, and add on top black raspberries, strawberries, leafy spinach, top off with slices of banana. And believe me, it's good. It's a really fulfilling breakfast.

I used to drink black coffee in the morning to help me with most of my joint pain because of some compounds it carries, like antioxidants and anti-inflammatory properties that fight free radicals and inflammation. I'm not saying coffee is a cure, I am just saying it was helping me as one of my personal home remedies. It might not work for everyone. But for me, that black coffee in the morning was essential.

Why black coffee specifically? Because adding milk or cream or sugar changes the compounds. Black coffee has chlorogenic acids that reduce inflammation. It has polyphenols that fight oxidative stress. And the warmth of it helps loosen up my stiff joints in the morning. I'd wrap my hands around that hot mug and feel my fingers start to relax. I'd take that first sip and feel the warmth travel down into my chest, into my stomach, and somehow it would make the aching in my legs and ankles a little more bearable.

I started noticing that certain foods and soft drinks or hot beverages would help certain medical issues in the body, like lowering high blood pressure or sleeping disorders or bloating of the stomach. I would also take natural foods and over the counter vitamins to also get my day started, like Men's One A Day multivitamin, or I'll make myself a banana and orange juice smoothie, or I'll eat a medium size bowl full of mixed grapes and mixed berries with slices of watermelon and apples.

Here's my exact weekly breakdown:

I try to eat six pomegranate seed servings a month. I eat ten steamed carrots three times a week to keep my eyesight on point. I eat two baked sweet potatoes a week. I eat baked wild caught salmon smothered with mushrooms three times a week. I eat a small portion of turkey breast baked in the oven once a week. I do the same with small white chicken thighs. And I eat one portion of T-bone steak a month.

All these different foods I just named provide me with essential nutrients like high quality proteins, stuff like iron, zinc, and vitamin B12, which support my muscle, bone, and metabolic health, which is very important for people living with lupus!

The way I do my boost of proteins and vitamins, I break everything down on a certain day of the week and month so my body will not get immune to it. Because if your body gets immune to any medications, to any type of proteins, or to a home remedy, you will not feel the difference between the time you felt normal energized to a boosted up energized.

And once you don't feel the difference, you will either do two things that can harm you in the long term. One is you will either go much more extra on your over-the-counter vitamins, or go extra on the beef and meat. And both can make you have too much iron and calcium, which is bad for people living with lupus.

That's why I rotate. That's why I break it down by day and week and month. Carrots on Monday, Wednesday, Friday. Salmon on Tuesday, Thursday, Saturday. Turkey once a week. Steak once a month. My body never gets used to any one thing, so everything stays effective.

I would make daily lists to stay on track with my diet and routine. I had too much going on that I would actually forget about my number one mission I was supposed to get done for that day of the week. So I had to keep a mini notepad on me on what to take care of first. And everything I had written down had a time zone and time limits, so I would take every mission seriously.

I try to keep my schedule with how all the ways I do my meals, like I do my days, with what I got to do on my to do list. Like a typical day for me is I will get up around 4:00 AM and drink a glass of hot water with lemon. And then eat either fruits or a smoothie while taking my medications. I'll see what bills have to be paid for that week or month. I'll look around my house to see if anything is running short with my food and cosmetics.

Here's what a typical to do list looks like for me:

4:00 AM: Wake up, hot water with lemon.

4:30 AM: Medications with fruit or smoothie.

5:00 AM: Wound care, 1.5 to 2 hours.

7:00 AM: Black coffee, vitamin booster snack.

8:00 AM, Check bills, make calls if needed.

9:00 AM: Supermarket or farmer's market.

12:00 PM: Come home, cook, clean.

2:00 PM: Rest period, if needed.

3:00 PM: Exercise bike, meditation.

4:00 PM: Research, reading, projects.

6:00 PM: Dinner.

8:00 PM: TV and relaxation.

9:00 PM: Prepare for next day, check tomorrow's list.

10:00 PM: Bed.

Everything on that list has a time, and everything has a purpose. And I stick to it as much as my body will let me.

In the mornings I go through my things, see what I need and then I go straight to the supermarket and farmers market, taking my time, admiring the scenery, the colors of the flowers and fruits and vegetables, and the people who are doing the same thing as me. Then I'll go on the highway for a nice drive while listening to my favorite music. I spend about three hours of outside time enjoying myself, exploring different supermarkets and clothing stores. And then I'll come back home. So within

That three-hour morning routine? That's my therapy. That's my peace. That's when I feel most normal, most human, most like Johnny instead of just "the guy with lupus." Walking through the produce section, touching the fruits, smelling the fresh flowers, that's healing that no doctor can prescribe.

I'll start cooking and cleaning and then watch one hour of TV, and I'll read a book at the same time, doing research on my new ideas and projects I'm working on for the future. Then I'll get on my exercising bike and meditate and concentrate as I work out. I do this every day, sometimes twice a day.

There were times I couldn't complete a day of my missions because my body just didn't feel up to it, especially when the weather is bad outside. Like rain. Or snowing. Or if it's really cold out. Certain weather conditions make my lupus very active. Either my joints are in pain, my arthritis is active, my legs and toes will swell up and get numb.

And when everything is hurting me like that, I'll just do what I can do from my home to do list. I'll check my bills list, see what's due, and make some phone calls to bypass some time. I prioritize. If I can't go out, I handle what I can from home. If I can't stand long enough to cook a big meal, I make something simple. Like my go-to comfort mean; my famous bakes chicken soup.

I like to bake my chicken soup. It just brings out the flavor much better. I'll chop up potatoes and carrots, celery, onion and green pepper, and add the small Cornish hen chicken, and put some whole garlic cloves. And let it cook on top of the stove for about an hour. Then slide it in the oven with the top lid on the pot, so it's like a smothered bake cooking style. I'll let that bake slow for two hours with the oven heated at 250 degrees, and that baked chicken soup is to die for.

That's my comfort meal on some bad days. The smell of it cooking fills the house, and even though I'm hurting, even though I can't leave my house, even though I can barely walk, at least I can make myself something good to eat. At least I can still take care of myself when it comes down to preparing myself a good meal that way I am still ahead of the game of knowing I am still alive in some normal fields.

I can remember in 2009, I lived on my couch and it was a struggle to get around. I couldn't even leave my bed

and both my legs had a lot of open sores. I was so depressed and stressed out because I had no help at that
time.

I had a small table next to my couch, and it had all my
meds and waters and snacks. Everything I needed was
within arm's reach because I couldn't walk to get it. Not
that good anyways. The couch became my bed, my din-
ing table became my office, so where the couch was in
my living room became my world. For a nice amount of
time. I had my companion at the time who was a female
red nosed, light brown pit bull.

My dog was like an angel that I believe was sent by God
to help me cope with my pain and suffering. She stayed
by my side the whole time. When I was moaning from
the pain, my dog would try licking my face or licking
my legs where the pain was, trying to help ease it. She
definitely had been and was truly a blessing from God.

During the time I couldn't get out of bed, which was my
couch at the time, my dog would stay by my side until
my girlfriend came home from work. She worked 9 to
5. And when she came home, she'd help out, especially
getting me off the couch and up and around to the bathroom to bathe and get dressed and getting undressed,
and organizing my medications.

I went through that routine for about five months until
my legs started feeling better and my wounds were
closing a little, enough so I could stand up and walk
around my house a little bit to do for myself.

Five months. That's the longest period I couldn't leave
my bed. Five months of living on a couch. Five months

of depending on my dog and my girlfriend for everything. Five months of wondering if this was my life now, if this was all I had left.

At that time I was going through a dark, painful moment, and what got me through was God letting me still wake up in the morning to see another day, to live life no matter what my situation was like. What got me through was still being able to enjoy playing with my dog and seeing my grandkids and having the support of my girlfriend.

That's what got me through the really dark days when the pain is unbearable. It's not the medication. It's not the doctors. It's the small moments. It's your dog licking your face. It's your grandkids' laughter. It's your girlfriend coming home from work and helping you to the bathroom without making you feel like a burden. It's waking up in the morning and realizing you made it through another night.

It's knowing that even though you're living on a couch with open sores on your legs and you can't walk and you can't work and you can't do most of the things you used to do, you're still here. You're still alive. You're still fighting.

And as long as you're still here, there's hope. As long as you're still breathing, there is a chance that things can get better. As long as you're still praying, God is still listening.

That's what gets me through. That's what pulled me off that couch after five months. That's what gets me out of bed every morning even when it takes fifteen to twenty minutes just to sit up.

Faith. Family. And the refusal to give up.

Chapter 6
Mastering My Financial Issues

It is now time to master my financial issues. And I'm going to master them like when I'm in the kitchen chefing it up with my seasonings and special spices.

Because here's the truth: if you don't have fun making money, you will stop striving so hard. You'll lose that entrepreneur state of mind. You'll stop being willing to try anything that can bring you money.

It's definitely all about that strong state of mindset. That mindset is what gets you through the hardest struggles of your life. Especially when you're battling a chronic disease. Especially when you're dealing with disappointments from family, friends, and relationships.

Listen, making money when you're sick is like cooking a good meal. You got to have the right ingredients. You got to know how to mix them together. You got to season it just right. And you got to have fun doing it, or else the whole thing falls apart. There are two sides to the world, whether you want to believe it or not.

I started figuring things out from my own experience. When you're suffering with an illness you'll be living with for most of your life, and that illness is always bringing pain to the sensitive parts of your body, it changes everything. Oh yes indeed it changes everything and I mean the headaches that turn into migraines, stomachaches that turn into stomach ulcers, varicose veins in your legs that turn into leg ulcers, and toes that go numb when you stand too long, walk too far or travel too much.

You yourself, or anybody else, just wouldn't want to put themselves through that most of the time. So it becomes another reason to give up on yourself. Another excuse to quit trying to live a better life.

Having people around you who are healthy also changes thing. You see them having no type of medical issues that they have to struggle with every day like some of us battling our illness 24 hours a day, 7 days a week. It's like our pain and suffering never stops, never stops giving us a hard time to cope with life. It's always on our mind, never letting us forget that we are suffering with an illness, and that chronic diseases can't be cured, only treated just to keep you alive to keep on suffering. Now isn't that something to think about people, did you hear what I just said, I said people who are suffering with any type of chronic illness, that's uncurable and only can just be treated with medications that can keep them alive, just to keep them suffering.

And I'm always wondering to myself how blessed most of these people are. They got a nine to five job. They have no worries. They don't have a clue what it's like for individuals living on the other side of the suffering world. That's right. I said it, suffering world.

So yes, there are two sides to this world.

On one side, you got people who have no worries in the world; those who can just get up in the morning and get going to their nine to five, do their daily routine with no health issues that will interfere. The only thing on their mind is: get that money, hang out with friends, buy expensive clothes, get a nice car.

They don't think about pain. They don't think about medication. They don't think about whether their body will let them make it through the day. They just live.

And then you have my side. The cold hearted, the vicious war. A person who always has to come up with ways to defeat my health issues to make it through the day. Yes, and I am talking all day every day.

My side, we have to think about every single move before we make it.

Every morning I wake up thinking: How am I going to make it through today? Is my lupus going to give me a hard time? Is it going to be very active? Will my legs be in more pain today than yesterday?

I'm always wondering if I even want to deal with the pain and suffering today. Wondering if I should put up with always having to sit down to take a break because I'm out of breath so quickly. Because my body is in so much pain.

I got to take off my shoes and socks to check my open wounds. See how badly they're leaking pus and blood. Check how swollen my legs and toes are.

If it's not too bad, I'll try to hang in there a little longer. If it doesn't look good, I have to cut my day very short. Get back home. Prepare myself for healing. Take my medications. Lay down.

And then start wondering: How am I going to make the next few dollars to pay my bills?

Oh, how I wish I was in that position where I didn't have to worry about situations like this.

Yes, it becomes very, very stressful.

So let me tell you about my monthly budget. I have to make $900 work for the rest of the month.

I lived in a studio apartment that I rented for $500 a month. Gas and electric included. I'm on SSI, receiving only $900 a month.

So after paying rent, I have about $400 left.

That $400 has to cover me until next month, like with my food shopping, cosmetics, underclothes, laundry, and my Wi Fi, which is $30 a month.

I spend about $100 on food and soft drink beverages. And I put up the rest of my money for emergencies. Like if I have to catch a cab somewhere far.

Let me show you how I stretch the $900 I receives a month after paying my $500 rent and having only $400 left over. So I use $30 for my wi-fi and a $100 for my food. So $100 worth of food can last me most of the month.

The remaining $270 has to cover my toiletries, under-clothes and laundry, emergency transportation fare, medical copays and anything unexpected. And when you have lupus, trust me, unexpected things come up all the time.

The type of money I really need to make a month to survive? At least $2,000 a month. And that's just to live in a low-income community. Not luxury. Not comfort. Just survival.

So every month, I'm $1,100 short.

$900 coming in, $2,000 needed. That's an $1,100 gap I got to fill every single month.

That's why I had no choice but to become a master en-trepreneur. I had to figure out ways to make that money. Because that $900 alone? It's just not enough. Not even close.

So I have to multiple side hustles going. And when you add them all up, they help me get closer to that $2,000 I need each month.

And you know what? As time goes on, when you got multiple hustles down packed, you can start to think of it like a nine to five. You start to feel like you're back in the normal world with everybody else.

One of my most profitable side hustles is selling food.

I'm known more for my cooking more than my barbering even though I've been cutting hair on the side way before getting my Master Barber License. And the people who know my food were the people who love my food. Because of the experience of my cooking in the path before suffering with lupus, I was well known to as a chef in many restaurants.

So as I was selling food on the weekend, once a month, and it was bringing me about $300 to $400. And I'm only doing it for a couple hours. Like three hours of selling food.

Think about that. Three hours. $300 to $400. That's more than I get from the government in a whole week.

That's the power of using your skills. That's why I say you got to chef up your money like you chef up your meals. You season it right. You make it taste good. You make people want to come back for more.

When I couldn't pay rent, I remember I needed $300, and $300 I DID not have one time.

At times I couldn't pay any bills but rent. And sometimes, I couldn't even pay that.

I remember one time specifically. Rent was due. I had $200 to my name. That's it. $200.

Rent was $500.

I was $300 short. And I didn't know where that money was going to come from.

I called my landlord. Told him the truth. I said, "Listen, I am short a little this month on rent, am not working to much lately because I am suffering with lupus. And it is very active right now, and besides that I can't really work a regular job at this time I got $200 right now. Can I pay you that for now and give you the rest in two weeks once I receive the rest of my money?"

You know what he said?

"No. Rent is due on the first. And you know this shit, dammit. If you can't pay, you got to go my man, I am not trying to have these types of problems and I'm sorry I have nothing to do with you suffering with lupus, please don't start putting that on me. "

I said hell no man, my lupus is my problem.

And just like that he told me, "I have no compassion for you, I have no understanding of this disease you're suffering from. So I am saying, you just have to go. "

So I had to swallow my pride. I had to call a friend. And I had to ask for help. And once the rest of my money came through, I was able to pay back the friend I borrowed from.

I was so blessed to have a friend at that time to loan me the money and I wasted no time to pay it back.

But that feeling? That feeling of having to ask? That feeling of not knowing if I'd have a roof over my head? That stays with you.

That's why I hustle the way I hustle now. Because I never want to be in that position again. I never want to have to borrow money off of a friend or anyone just to keep a roof over my head. Choosing between medications, food, or paying bills is a choice no one should have to make.

I remember when I had to pay a portion for my medications. And one time, I couldn't do it.

So here's what I did. If I had enough meds to hold me until my next doctor's visit, I'd pass up getting that refill. I'd stretch the meds I already had.

How do you stretch medication?

You skip a day or two. You skip a dose. If your meds say take twice a day, you only take it once a day. Or you cut the tablet in half to help stretch the time. It was something I had to do until I was approved for some help by some health insurance.

Let me paint you the picture of what that looks like in real life.

You're standing at the pharmacy counter. The pharmacist tells you your medication is $50 for the month.

You look in your wallet. You got $75 to your name but you still need to buy food, still need to do laundry, still need to get to your next doctor's appointment.

So you make a choice. You tell the pharmacist, "I'll come back for it next week."

You walk out with that $75 still in your pocket. You go to the grocery store. You buy the cheapest food you can find; rice, chicken. The basics.

You go home. You take the medication bottle you still have from last month. And you cut those pills in half.

The bottle says, "Take two pills twice a day."

But you take one pill once a day.

Because you have to make it stretch. You got to make it last until you can afford to refill it.

And while you're doing that, you're praying. Praying that cutting the dose in half won't make your lupus flare up. Praying you can make it through the next two weeks without a major problem. Praying your body can handle the reduced medication.

That's the choice people with chronic illness face every single day.

Medication or food. Medication or rent. Medication or transportation to the doctor who prescribes the medication.

It's a cycle. It's a trap. And it's the reality for millions of people in this country. And this is how I saved money.

It takes a lot of discipline to keep your mind focused on doing better for yourself helps. I try to never get caught up spending extra money on things I really don't need.

I try to be really disciplined with myself. Once I get all my real important needs out of the way, I put my leftover money away. Just as simple as that.

Here's my system, and it works:

First priority: Rent gets paid. No matter what the situation is, because without a roof over your head, you have nothing.

Second priority: wi-fi gets paid. I need internet to research help resources, to find ways to make money and to hustle online.

Third priority: food gets bought. But I shop smart. I buy in bulk when things are on sale. I cook at home. I don't eat out. I make meals that stretch over multiple days. But not too many days, 2 days max. Rice and beans. Chicken and vegetables. Soup that lasts for days.

Fourth priority: Emergency fund. Whatever is left over, even if it's just $20, it goes into my emergency stash. Because emergencies always come when you least expect them.

And here's what I don't do: I don't buy things I don't need.

I don't buy new clothes unless it's a special engagement of a kind. If my old ones kept up well, I don't buy the latest phone. I don't buy expensive shoes. I wear what

I got until it doesn't fit well anymore or it's not wearable.

That's discipline. That's how you survive on a $900 a month. You prioritize. You sacrifice. You save every single penny you can. I know that's to impossible but you have to try.

Let me tell you having help from the government, especially trying to apply for SSI, it was a struggle. A real battle to get approved to receive help from them.

Because they will turn you down so many times that it'll make you want to just give up. Getting help is tough. From any federal government.

Let me tell you how that process works.

You apply for SSI SSD. You fill out all the paperwork. Every single page. You get all your medical records together. You get letters from your doctors explaining your condition. You submit everything. And then you wait. Most times the wait is a year or two.

And then you get a letter in the mail. Saying you've been denied. So you appeal. You get more documentation. You get more letters from more doctors. You explain in detail how lupus affects your daily life. How you can't work a regular job. How you need help just to survive.

You submit everything again. And you wait again.

Another letter comes. Saying you are denied again.

So you appeal a third time. And this time, you might need to get a lawyer to help you. And you go through the whole process all over again. More paperwork. More waiting. More stress piling on top of the stress of lupus.

And they keep turning you down. Over and over. Until you start thinking, "Maybe I don't deserve help. Maybe I should just give up. Maybe I should just figure it out on my own."

And that's exactly what they want. They want you to give up. Because if you give up, they don't have to pay you. It's a strategy. Deny, deny, deny until people stop trying.

But I didn't give up.

I kept fighting. I kept appealing. And finally, after two years, I got approved.

Two years.

That's how long it took. Two years of struggling even worse than I had to. Two years of not knowing how I'd pay my bills. Two years of stress on top of stress.

But I made it through. And that $900 a month? It isn't much. But it's something. It's a foundation. It's a starting point to build from.

But with financial issues, it was stressful trying to maintain a relationship.

It's tough not knowing what's going to happen with you and your girlfriend, or wife. It can be depressing. Because financial issues can cause a breakup. They can separate even a happy couple.

Let me tell you how this works in real life.

You're with someone you love. Someone who supports you. Someone who understands your lupus and stands by you through the pain.

But you can't take her out on special occasions because you don't have the money.

You can't buy her the birthday gift that you know she will want and love because you got to save that money for medication.

You can't go on trips or take vacations because you barely have enough for rent.

And she says she understands. And maybe she really does.

But it still weighs on you. It still sits heavy on your chest. It still makes you feel like less of a man.

You wonder if she'd be better off with someone who can provide for her. Someone who can take care of her. Someone who doesn't have to choose between medication and taking her to see a movie.

And the stress of that? The weight of that? It can break relationships.

Not because the love isn't there. But because poverty and chronic illness are heavy burdens to carry. And sometimes, two people just can't carry them together.

I was BLESSED. My girlfriend, my fiancée, she stuck with me. She understood. She supported me. She never made me feel bad about not having money. She never complained. She never pressured me.

She saw me for who I was, not for what I could buy her.

But I know a lot of people who weren't that blessed. I know relationships that ended because the financial stress was just too much. Because one person got tired of struggling. Because the bills piled up and the love couldn't survive under all that pressure.

That's why financial freedom isn't just about money. It's about relationships. It's about not having to stress about bills when you should be enjoying time with the person you love. It's about being able to take care of the people who take care of you.

And my advice to someone who's living with any type of chronic disease. If you can't work a traditional job, don't just sit there feeling sorry for yourself.

Grab anything you can get your hands on. The internet. A desktop computer. A laptop. Your phone. Or go to a library in your neighborhood that lets you use their computers.

Do your research on help resources in your town, your county, your state, your country. The help is out there. But you got to look for it.

Look for:

Government assistance programs: SSI, SSD, food stamps, Medicaid, housing assistance.

Grants specifically for people with chronic illness.

Nonprofit organizations that help with medical bills, rent, and utilities.

Community resources like food banks, free clinics, and transportation services.

Online ways to make money: freelancing, selling things you make, offering services you can do from home.

It's all out there. I promise you, it's out there.

But nobody's going to come knock on your door and hand it to you. You got to go find it. You got to put in the work. Even when you're tired. Even when you're in pain. Even when you want to give up.

Because the alternative? The alternative is sitting there watching the bills pile up while your situation gets worse and worse.

I know it's hard. I know you're exhausted. I know your body hurts. But you got to fight. You got to hustle. You got to find a way.

My dream is to one day accomplish financial freedom.

If I can get my own restaurant or barbershop and be successful with my business in the future, that's what financial freedom looks like to me.

It means I can call my own shots in life. I can pick my own time to have fun and enjoy myself. I don't have to wait on some miracle money to just pop up. I don't have to wish for a winning lottery ticket.

I want to be in control of my destiny. My future. My time living on this earth. That is financial freedom to me.

And my dream number? My goal?

To see a couple million one day.

Let me paint you a picture of what financial freedom really means:

It's waking up in the morning and not worrying about bills. Not worrying if I got enough money for medication. Not worrying if I can afford to eat the healthy food that keeps my lupus under control.

It's owning my own barbershop slash restaurant. The one I've been dreaming about. Where people can come get a fresh haircut on one side and get a good meal on the other side.

Where I'm the boss. Where I control of the hours. Where I can sit down when I need to sit. Where I can rest when I need to rest. Where I don't have to explain my lupus to anybody or ask permission to take care of my health.

It's being able to take my fiancée on a real vacation. Somewhere nice. Somewhere she can relax and not worry. Somewhere we can enjoy each other without the stress of money hanging over us.

It's being able to help other people who are struggling the way I struggled. Being able to give somebody a loan when they're short on rent without worrying about how I'll pay my own bills. Being able to be the friend to someone else that my friend was to me.

It's seeing a couple million in the bank one day. Not to be flashy. Not to buy expensive cars or designer clothes. But to have security. To have peace of mind.

To know that no matter what happens with my lupus, no matter how bad it gets, I'll be okay. I'll be taken care of. I won't ever have to choose between medication and food again.

That's financial freedom. That's what I'm working toward. That's what keeps me hustling even on the days when my body is screaming at me to stop.

Because I refuse to be poor and sick for the rest of my life. I refuse to let lupus steal my dreams along with my health. I refuse to give up.

Because it's nothing worse than always having to think about how you're going to make it in the world as times change.

Especially with new mayors and governors and presidents. They keep getting tougher on laws. They keep requiring more certifications. To get a driver's license. To get certain degrees to operate a business. To meet certain criteria to be employed for certain jobs.

The people running this world make it tough and rough for the unfortunate. For the disabled. For the elderly. Especially if you got a family with young adults and minors depending on you.

If parents can't take care of their young children, those kids fall into the streets and into self-destruction. And that's why there's so many brutal crimes happening in today's world.

They keep making the rules harder. More requirements. More certifications. More hoops to jump through.

And when you got a chronic illness, you can't jump through hoops. Some days you can barely stand up.

But they don't care. They don't see you as a person. They see you as a number. As a liability. As someone who's going to cost them money.

So they make the process longer. They make the denials more frequent. They hope you'll give up. They hope you'll just disappear.

But we can't give up. We can't disappear.

Because if we do, nothing changes. If we do, they win.

So we fight. We hustle. We find ways to survive despite the system working against us. We support each other. We share resources. We lift each other up.

Because that's what being a master entrepreneur really means when you got a chronic illness. It's not just about making money. It's about mastering your situation. It's about refusing to let the world break you. It's about finding ways to thrive even when the system is designed to make you fail.

That's what this chapter is about. That's what my whole life is about.

Mastering my financial issues so that lupus doesn't get to master me.

Chapter 7
The Music That Got Me Through Most of These Challenges in My Life

To me, and this is my own opinion, my own beliefs, my own experience, music holds so much healing power.

To the mind. To the body itself.

Like I said before, lupus is my problem. People who know about it, people who know someone with it, family or friend, people living with lupus have pain throughout the whole body.

That's just the reality of this disease. Pain everywhere. All the time. You also even get tired of

The problem with the medications I took were that they had side effects, and sometimes those side effects are worse than the disease itself.

So I used to try home remedies. Yes, they gave me some comfort. Yes, the pain came to some ease.

But most of the home remedies and prescriptions always had a backend. Some sort of side effects. If it didn't make me itch like crazy and break out in hives, it made me sleep all throughout the day. If it didn't make me sleep all day, it made my stomach hurt. Gave me stomach ulcers. If it didn't tear up my stomach, it made my body swell up in some parts.

There was always something.

The medications that helped with joint pain? They made me itch so bad I'd scratch my skin raw. Break out in hives all over my arm and chest. I'd be sitting there trying not to scratch but I couldn't help it. The itch was maddening.

The medications that helped with inflammation? They knocked me out cold. Made me sleep all most of my day away. I'd wake up feeling drugged. Feeling like I'd lost whole days of my life. Like I was sleeping my life away. And most of

The medications that helped with the lupus itself? They tore up my stomach. Gave me stomach ulcers that burned like fire. Made me throw up. Made me afraid to eat because I knew the pain was coming the minute food hit my stomach.

And almost all of them made me swell up. My face would puff up. My hands would swell so big I couldn't make a fist. My legs would get bigger and bigger. I'd look in the mirror and not recognize myself.

So I used to stress to myself. "What is going on? What is it going to take to improve my situation with lupus and the pain that it brings to me?"

There's got to be something better than this. There's got to be a way to manage the pain without destroying something else in my body.

I said, "Let me try working out a bit. And let me listen to some of my favorite music while I do it."

I didn't know it then, but that simple decision changed everything.

It was July 21, 2010, the day God spoke to me through song; my birthday. I was feeling good and happy I had made it to another year.

I was sitting in my house on the couch. And I was rocking back and forward. Moaning in pain. But still happy although I was in pain,

The lupus was hitting me hard that day. My whole body ached. My joints felt like they were on fire. Every muscle hurt. Every bone hurt. I couldn't get comfortable no matter how I positioned myself.

I'd try sitting up. Too much pain. I'd try lying down. Too much pain. I'd try leaning to the left. To the right. Nothing helped.

So I just rocked. Back and forward. Back and forward. Moaning in pain.

That's where I was on my birthday. Not celebrating. Not with family. Not eating cake. Just alone on my couch. Rocking. Moaning. Suffering. But still happy.

And then a song came on the radio.

By Earth, Wind, and Fire. The song was called

"The Reasons."

And I stopped rocking. Because it did something to my mind, it caught my attention to where my mind froze, taking my mind off of the pain, and just thinking how smooth this song was by the words that was matching the situation that was going on in my life at the time.

I figured God wanted me to hear that particular song for a reason. And the reasons why I say that? Because the song had me thinking. "I guess the reasons why I am here now in this position is to change my lifestyle."

I believe God put lupus in my life for so many reasons because of all the wrong choices in was making in life my mother kept warning me about or

Maybe because I wasn't eating the right foods. All that fried food. All that processed food. All that junk I was putting in my body.

Maybe because I wasn't going to church on a regular basis. I'd gotten lazy with my faith. I gotten to Comfortable and not Taking God for granted.

Maybe because I was getting too comfortable hanging out with the wrong group of friends. The ones my mom warned me about. The ones who weren't taking me anywhere good in life only to a future of self-destruction and disaster.

So now, after that song went off, another one came on.

By the same artist. It was called Keep Your Head to the Sky. It seemed like a sign from God. I was not sure, but it was starting to do something for me.

And all I could think about was: God is speaking to me. Right now. Through these songs.

He's saying, "Now that your life is about to change for the best for you, stop crying in pain!"

"Soak it up and keep your head up to the sky."

"Be ready for your blessings that's about to come your way."

"It's all you can do right now."

That birthday. That moment on the couch. Those two songs back-to-back. That's when I discovered music could be some sort of home remedy for natural healing.

And the reason why I believe I like Earth, Wind and Fire specifically is because my mom use to listen to it when I was a child in the '70s. So it kind of brings back good memories.

Good memories of being young and healthy. Running around the house with no pain. No swollen legs. No open wounds. Just being a kid.

Good memories of family gatherings. And all of my aunts, uncles and cousins everywhere. Music playing loud. People dancing. People laughing.

Good memories of my mom dancing in the living room. Me, my brothers and sisters, everyone either dancing or trying to sing the song.

Good memories of a times before lupus. Before pain. Before struggle. Before everything got hard.

When I hear Earth Wind and Fire, I don't just hear music.

I hear my childhood.

I hear love.

I hear hope.

I hear possibility.

And there's something about their sound. The horns. The harmonies. The uplifting messages in the lyrics.

The way the music makes you want to move even when your body hurts.

The way it lifts your spirit even when you're depressed.

It's like the music was made for healing. Like God designed these songs specifically to reach down into your soul and pull you up when you're at your lowest.

So that's when I started to make myself a healing playlist of all these songs I used to listen to when I was in pain, and they got me through most of the times, were:

Earth Wind and Fire: "The Reasons" "Keep Your Head to the Sky" "Devotion"

These three songs became my foundation. My medicine. My therapy.

Now there was another artist that helped me also. The Isley Brothers.

The Isley Brothers: "At Your Best (You Are Love)" "Here We Go Again" "Footsteps in the Dark"

Then another one of my favorite artists. The Stylistics.

The Stylistics: "Betcha by Golly, Wow," "People Make the World Go Around" "You Are Everything" "Children of the Night"

And yes, so it's like all my favorite music artist songs were just coming on. In the order I would play them.

This artist is called Blue Magic.

Blue Magic: "Just Don't Want to Be Lonely" "Stop to Start" "Chasing Rainbows" "What's Come Over Me"

So there it is; one of my completed playlists to help me when I was in pain and feeling in a depressed mood.

It really got me through. And yes

Of course, there are plenty of other songs. But these are the exact ones from that specific day. That birthday, July 21, 2010.

And then my daily soundtrack started to expand:

The Stylistics, Blue Magic, Chic (One of my favorite songs: "I Want Your Love") All songs by The Isley Brothers, Marvin Gaye, Bob Marley and Smokey Robinson.

Most music from that era, within that time frame, from the '70s and '80s, helped me get through some of the tough times of my journey living with lupus. I was so blessed to discover how music physically changes my pain, helps me with my stretching, my pushup. It gave me some type of freedom.

So I put on some old classic Earth Wind and Fire.

In this order: "Keep Your Head to the Sky" "Devotion" "The Reasons"

It seemed like the music was meant to be played in that order.

Because the music was hitting in all the right places for me.

Let me explain what happened. How music physically changed my pain.

Song one: "Keep Your Head to the Sky"

As the song started playing, I was spreading my arms wide, looking up at the sky, stretching as I prayed to myself, "It's got to be a better way, God. There's got to be a better way to deal with my situation living with lupus."

And as I stretched, something happened.

I could feel my muscles loosening. The tightness in my shoulders easing. The stiffness in my back releasing.

It was like the music was giving me permission to move.

Like it was telling my body, "You can do this. You can stretch through the pain. You can move. You're not as broken as you think."

Song Two: "Devotion"

And as the song Devotion came on, I started doing pushups.

Saying to myself, "I definitely got to start devoting some time to working out all the time."

"Because it's really making my body feel much better. I'm feeling much healthier. And it lasts all day."

The music was fueling me. Giving me energy I didn't know I had.

Each beat of the drums was like fuel for another pushup.

Each horn blast was like a coach yelling, "One more! You can do one more!"

And the pain was still there. Don't get me wrong.

But it was like the music was louder than the pain.

Like it was drowning out the voice in my head that was saying, "Stop. You can't do this. You're too sick. You're too weak. Lay back down. Give up."

The music was louder. And I kept going on with my life.

Song Three: "The Reasons"

And as the song The Reasons started playing, all I could keep saying to myself was:

"It must have been a reason why God led me to start playing music."

"And a reason for me to try working out."

"This is it. This is the answer I've been looking for."

I started feeling so good.

Like I was free of all pain and stress.

Like the lupus had taken a break. Like it had left my body for a minute.

Like my body was mine again. Like I was in control instead of the disease being in control.

Those songs helped ease my mind.

They made me stop dwelling on my pain.

And start thinking about what I am going to start doing to deal with it.

Knowing pain will be part of my life situations now. Knowing I'll have to deal with it every now and then.

But also knowing I have a weapon now. Music. God gave me music.

Different pain needed different music.

I learned this through trial and error. Through paying attention to my body. Through listening to what helped and what didn't. And

If I had a migraine, I'd listen to a much softer type of music from my playlist.

Something smooth. Something gentle. Something that wouldn't aggravate the pounding in my head.

Songs like: The Stylistics, "Betcha by Golly, Wow" Smokey Robinson, soft ballads Marvin Gaye, "What's Going On"

These songs are slow. Calm. They don't have loud drums or blaring horns.

They ease into your mind like a cool cloth on a hot forehead.

They quiet the noise. They soften the pain.

When I have a migraine, my head feels like it's splitting open. Light hurts. Sound hurts. Movement hurts. Everything hurts.

So I need music that soothes instead of stimulates. Music that whispers instead of shouts. Music that rocks me gently instead of pumping me up.

If my arthritis started acting up, I would play upbeat music that forced me to move. Something with energy. Something with movement. Something that made me want to fight through the stiffness.

Songs like: Earth Wind and Fire, "Keep Your Head to the Sky" Chic, "I Want Your Love" The Isley Brothers, "Here We Go Again"

These songs have energy. They have beat. They have drive.

They make you want to move even when your joints are screaming at you not to.

They give you the motivation to push through. To do your stretches. To do your exercises. To keep your body from locking up completely.

When my arthritis acts up, everything gets stiff. My fingers. My knees. My elbows. My back. Everything.

And if I don't move, it gets worse. The stiffness turns into immobility. The pain gets deeper. The joints lock up. So I needed music that forces me to move. That gives me the energy to fight through the pain and keep my joints working. Am surprised some of the

I shared some music with two of my doctors in the past. And I told them, "When I try to level out the pain, instead of always taking meds for the pain, I try listening to my favorite music."

One of the doctors looked at me surprised. He said, "That's really good, Johnny. That's actually really good."

I said, "The sound of music helps me keep my mind off the pain. And it helps with my situations I am going through with lupus. It's like natural therapy. It doesn't have side effects. It doesn't make me sick. It just makes me feel better."

My doctor said, "I never thought of that type of treatment."

He paused. Then he said, "That's actually brilliant. Music therapy is a real thing. We use it in hospitals for cancer patients. For people with Alzheimer's. For people with depression. But I never thought to recommend it for lupus patients."

And that made me realize something important.

I wasn't just finding ways to cope. I was discovering real medical treatment. Something doctors didn't even think to prescribe. Something that worked as well as medications. Without the side effects. Without the itching. Without the sleeping all day. Without the stomach ulcers.

Just healing. Pure healing.

And for my workouts, I used a certain type of music.

It's a must. Not optional. I can't work out without it.

I usually used music with hype to it. Like typical songs from the '70s and '80s.

I like this group called Chic and their song called I Want Your Love.

There's another song by a group called Zhané. And their song is called Hey Mr. DJ.

Let me tell you about one specific workout where music made all the difference. Where music made the impossible possible.

It was a really bad day. One of those days where lupus wins before you even get out of bed.

My legs were swollen. My joints were aching. I'd been in bed most of the morning because I just couldn't get my body to cooperate. And I knew I needed to work out. I knew I needed to move.

Because if I stayed in bed all day, I'd be even worse tomorrow. The stiffness would set in. The pain would get deeper. The lupus would get stronger.

But I had no energy. No motivation.

I was looking at my exercise bike thinking, "There's no way. I can't do this today. My body won't let me."

Then I put on my workout playlist.

And the first song that came on was "I Want Your Love" by Chic.

That bassline hit.

That funky, driving, unstoppable bassline.

And something in me woke up.

I got on the bike. Slowly. Painfully. But I got on.

And I started pedaling.

And at first, it hurt. My knees were stiff. My ankles were swollen. Every push of the pedal sent pain shooting up my legs.

But the music kept going. The beat kept pushing me. And I kept pedaling. By the time the song was halfway through, I wasn't thinking about the pain anymore. I was thinking about the rhythm. I was moving with the music. I was part of the song.

And then "Hey Mr. DJ" came on.

And that song is even more upbeat. Even more energy. Even more driving force.

And I was flying on that bike.

Pedaling faster than I'd pedaled in weeks. Feeling stronger than I'd felt in months.

By the time the workout was over, I'd done thirty minutes on the bike.

Thirty minutes!

On a day when I could barely get out of bed. On a day when I thought working out was impossible.

That's what music did for me. That's the power it has.

It can take you from "I can't" to "I did" in the span of two songs.

There are some songs that also make my symptoms worse, and most of those are rap songs.

Let me be clear, I'm not saying all rap is bad. There's conscious rap. There's rap with messages. There's rap that tells stories and speaks truth. That kind of rap I respect.

But the rap I'm talking about? The kind that has no purpose, no meanings. Those rap songs that just want to make noise and scream out curse words.

It drives me nuts.

I turn my radio station every time that kind of rap song comes on.

Because I can feel it physically. My heart rate goes up. My blood pressure rises. My stress levels spike.

And stress is one of the biggest lupus triggers.

Stress makes the inflammation worse. Makes the pain worse. Makes the swelling worse. Makes everything worse.

It's like my body reacts to negative music the same way it reacts to trigger foods. It attacks itself. The lupus gets more active. The symptoms get stronger.

So I stay away from it.

I protect my peace. I protect my health.

I only let music into my ears that lifts me up. That heals me. That helps me.

Life is hard enough with lupus. I don't need music making it harder.

And this is the reason why I create a playlist of my favorite songs.

It is a must.

This is how most of my projects gets done in a timely manner. This is how I stay focused. This is how I push through the pain and get things done anyway. Like my cooking playlist includes Marvin Gaye, Smokey Robinson and The Stylistics. Music that's smooth. That flows. That makes the kitchen feel like a sanctuary instead of a workplace.

When I'm cooking, I need music that matches the rhythm of chopping and stirring and seasoning. Music that makes the work feel like art instead of labor. Music that makes me want to take my time and do it right. Music that reminds me why I love cooking in the first place.

I also have my own barbering playlist that includes Earth, Wind and Fire, The Isley Brothers, Chic. Music with good vibes. Music that makes clients feel good. Music that creates the right atmosphere.

When I'm cutting hair, I need music that makes people relax. Music that makes conversation flow naturally. Music that makes the barbershop feel like community instead of just business. Music that says, "You're in good hands. Everything's going to be alright."

My exercise playlist has songs such as "I Want Your Love" by Chic, "Hey Mr. DJ" by Zhané, Earth Wind and Fire and similar upbeat songs. They have music with hype. Music with energy. Music that pushes me through the pain.

When I'm working out, I need music that forces me to move. Music that doesn't let me quit. Music that's louder than the voice in my head telling me to stop. Music that says, "One more. You can do one more." I also have

My own Pain Management Playlist: Earth Wind and Fire, "The Reasons," "Keep Your Head to the Sky," "Devotion" The Stylistics, "Betcha by Golly, Wow" Blue Magic, "Just Don't Want to Be Lonely"

Music that eases the mind. Music that speaks to the soul. Music that reminds me I'm not alone.

When I'm in pain, I need music that understands. Music that acknowledges the struggle but promises hope. Music that says, "I know it hurts. I know it's hard. But you're going to make it through. You always do." Now comes:

My Meditation Playlist: Bob Marley Smokey Robinson Soft instrumentals

Music that quiets the mind. Music that slows the breathing. Music that brings peace.

When I'm meditating or just trying to find some calm, I need music that creates space. Music that doesn't demand anything from me. Music that just lets me be. Music that says, "It's okay to rest. It's okay to be still. You don't have to fight right now."

And if I ever was in a position to meet these artists, I knew exactly what I'd say to them. I'd say, "Thank you.

Thank you for saving my life. At the time in need Because that's what you did. You saved my life when I was about to give up."

"When I was at my lowest, when I was rocking back and forth on my couch moaning in pain on my birthday, when I was ready to give up, again and again, when I couldn't see a way forward, your music reached out to me."

"You helped me cope with most of my health issues. Not just cope. Survive. Thrive."

"Your music gave me strength when my body had none. Your music gave me hope when I couldn't find it anywhere else. Your music gave me a reason to keep fighting when I wanted to quit."

"Your music helped me with faith. Faith in believing in myself. Faith that everything will be alright. Faith that no matter what I'm going through, I can keep my life moving."

"You probably made those songs decades ago. You probably don't even think about them anymore. You probably moved on to other projects, other albums, other stages of your life. You probably don't know that those songs are still working. Still healing. Still saving people."

"But they are. They're saving me. Every single day."

"So thank you. Thank you for the gift of music. Thank you for the gift of healing. Thank you for the gift of hope."

"You didn't just make music. You made medicine. And I'm living proof that it works."

Music became more than entertainment. It became treatment. It became therapy. It became survival.

When medications failed me, music didn't.

When doctors ran out of options, music gave me more.

When side effects made everything worse, music made everything better.

Music doesn't make me itch. Music doesn't make me sleep all day. Music doesn't give me stomach ulcers. Music doesn't make me swell up.

Music just heals.

It heals my body by getting me to move when I don't want to move. By getting me to stretch when I'm stiff. By getting me to exercise when I'm tired. By getting me off that couch when all I want to do is give up.

It heals my mind by taking me away from the pain. By giving me something to focus on besides lupus. By reminding me I'm more than my disease. By showing me I still have power even when my body is weak.

It heals my spirit by connecting me to my past. By bringing back memories of my mom dancing in the living room. By making me feel loved even when I'm alone. By reminding me who I was before lupus. And who I can still despite having it.

That's what music does for me. That's why this chapter matters. That's why I needed to tell you about it.

Because if you're reading this and you have lupus or any chronic illness, I want you to know something important:

There's more than medication. There is more than prescriptions. There is more than side effects that make you miserable.

There's music. And music heals.

Find your songs. Build your playlists. Let the music speak to you the way it spoke to me on July 21, 2010. On my birthday. On the day I was rocking back and forth in pain. On the day God decided to reach me through Earth, Wind and Fire.

Because somewhere in those melodies, somewhere in those lyrics, somewhere in those rhythms, you'll find what I found:

Hope.

Strength.

Healing.

And the courage to keep your head to the sky.

No matter how much it hurts. No matter how tired you are. No matter how many times you want to give up.

Keep your head to the sky.

Because the blessings are coming. God promised. Through the music, He promised.

And I believe Him.

Chapter 8:
How I Locked Down My Community With My Weekend Breakfast and Dinners

When I lived alone for two years, trying to come up with ways to earn some extra income while managing lupus, I started doing what came naturally to me. I cooked. Big breakfasts. Big dinners. And I shared them with my neighbors.

That's just who I am. That's what I do. It's how I was raised. My mother and grandmother taught me that when you have food, you share it. When people are hungry, you feed them. When your community is struggling, you help. Simple as that.

I was always offering plates to neighbors in my community. Just cook and share. Get to know people. Be familiar with your surroundings. Build connections. That's how you survive in a neighborhood. That's how you build family where blood isn't.

And they always gave me compliments on how good the food tasted.

"Man, Johnny, where'd you learn to cook like this?"

I'd smile and tell them about my mom. About working in restaurants from a young age. About learning that food is love made visible.

"Johnny, you need to sell this food. For real."

"This tastes better than most of these restaurants I eat at. I'd rather spend my money with you, bro. So what's good, Johnny, you think you want to do a little selling or what? Let me know and I'll pass word around the neighborhood. I'm well known over this way. This is where I grew up."

I'd just smile and say thank you. And I'd get right back to cooking. Even more than before now that I knew people were asking for it. Wanting it. Needing it.

And this all started on 157 Straight Street, Paterson, New Jersey. For two years, that neighborhood got excited that someone finally brought food cooked with love to their streets.

Let me paint you a picture of where I was living.

Most of the businesses around the area were run down. Nothing kept up well. Store owners didn't seem to care about keeping the fronts of their businesses clean. Food and snacks were outdated. You'd pick up a bag of chips, check the date, and it would be expired. I used to confirm it with the owner and they'd get mad and curse me out in a different language. I'm quite sure they were telling me to mind my own business. That I didn't have to buy anything if I didn't want to.

I'd say okay, no problem. And I'd leave.

It was a drug-infested area. Lots of crimes. Drug dealing going on everywhere. Abandoned factories and apartment buildings. You'd hear gunshots at night. See people running. See police lights flashing. That was just normal life in that neighborhood.

And every time we had big rainstorms, the area would flood.

The neighborhood was next to a river. When it rained hard, that river would overflow. Water would come rushing down the streets. Flooding up to people's houses and businesses. Some areas got flooded so bad that people were stuck in their houses for days. Business owners stuck in their places of work for days.

And the smell after was terrible.

Because after the floods, when the river started to recede, all the garbage from the river would be in the streets. Dead fish. Trash. Oil. Sewage. All mixed together. Rotting in the streets. And the turtles. Big turtles. The kind you see at Turtle Back Zoo. They'd been living in the river for years and would come out after the storms. You'd actually get to see the river's biggest creatures walking the streets, holding up traffic. Like an old Twilight Zone episode. Everyone standing around pointing and taking pictures while cops tried to direct the big turtles back into the river.

And you'd have homeless men and women out there trying to catch them. "Y'all crazy! You people better grab these turtles, they're good eating! You can make turtle stew or soup or fry them like steak!"

Man, some people were losing their minds watching homeless folks grab turtles and run down the street with them.

That's where I lived. And when I experienced those floods for the second time in a row, I knew I had to get myself together and get out from that neighborhood. But not yet. Not until I'd saved enough. Not until I'd figured out the next move.

So yes, every weekend I would cook big dinners.

Fried chicken. Baked turkey wings and rice with vegetables. I'd make a couple of aluminum trays. Big ones that could feed about twenty people.

And then I'd walk around the neighborhood offering food. To the homeless. To anyone who needed it.

I'd see them sitting on corners. Just hanging out, I guess doing what they do.

And I'd walk up. "Hey, you hungry? I got some food here."

And their eyes would light up. Like they couldn't believe someone was offering them a hot meal. A real meal. Not leftovers. Not scraps. But food I'd cooked fresh that morning.

"God bless you, brother."

"Thank you. Thank you so much."

"It's my pleasure to share my blessings, brother."

"Can I get two plates? For me and my friend?"

"Sure, why not? I cooked it to be eaten, not saved. I don't believe in having leftovers, brother. Take what you want and spread the word because good things don't last forever."

And I'd give them whatever they needed.

I did that same routine for a few weeks and months. Just cooking and giving. Gaining trust and respect within the community. Building my clientele. Not asking for anything back. Just feeding people who didn't mind a good home-cooked meal.

And let me tell you how word spread.

When neighbors started asking about the food, my homeboy from the neighborhood was running his mouth like a community news reporter. So yes, he was running his mouth, and soon other people in the neighborhood started asking about it.

At first, it was one neighbor. Miss Bridges, from down the street.

She stopped me one day. "Hi, is your name Johnny?"

"Yeah, why?"

"I've been watching you feed people every weekend. That food smells amazing. Can I buy a plate from you?"

I said, "You don't have to buy it. I'll give you a plate."

She said, "No, no. You're cooking all this food. Using your own money. Your own time. Let me pay you."

And she purchased a plate.

Then the next weekend, she came back with her sister. They both wanted plates. So they both purchased plates.

I was like, "Okay, thank you, and God bless you both."

And they said, "No, God bless you, young man, for bringing something we all can look forward to having on a weekend. Yes sir, nothing like a weekend dinner and movie."

I just laughed seeing an elderly church woman talk with some swagger.

Then the weekend after that, she came back with three friends.

And pretty soon, word was spreading. Not just in my neighborhood but other neighborhoods too. People were offering to pay me to cook whole spreads of food. For family get-togethers. For birthday parties. For Sunday after-church brunches.

And that's how I got into selling breakfasts and dinners on the weekends.

Now, every time I came outside to get my mail or start my journey, there were a few people waiting.

"Johnny, you cooking today?"

"Johnny, can I get a plate?"

"Johnny, my cousin's coming over, can you make extra?"

They were starting to be pests. But a good kind of pest. The kind that meant business was good.

So I officially started cooking and selling breakfast and dinners on the weekends. To earn a few dollars to help with my bills. And it was definitely good for me.

I'd still give out free food to the unfortunate. I definitely didn't stop and would never stop. That was part of who I was. Part of my purpose.

But if someone wanted something special cooked for a personal party, I would charge them a price. And I kept my prices fair. I wasn't trying to get rich. I was trying to pay my bills and help my community eat good food at the same time.

If a person wanted dinner cooked for ten to fifteen people and the food was in the chicken or meatloaf area, I'd charge them something very light. And if they wanted something from the turkey wings and oxtails or steaks area, I would charge them a fair amount but not nothing that they'd second guess. A price where they'd be like, "Oh wow, okay, I like that, thank you so much."

It especially depended on how much of a sale the supermarket would have that week. If chicken was on sale, I'd charge less. If oxtails were expensive that week,

I'd have to charge a little more. I was working with whatever the market gave me.

And this type of weekend hustle helped me a lot with my bills each month. That extra two hundred, three hundred, sometimes four hundred dollars on a good weekend? That made a big difference when paying off my bills each month and having a little left over to enjoy myself with.

And of course, you know after a while you have your individuals who will ask for some credit. Especially when they feel they've been supporting your business. And you know what, it's only right. Right?

It came a time when me and the neighbors were working together. I started giving credit for the dinners I made on Sundays only.

So every Sunday, I'd let it be known to the neighbors who used to purchase dinners on a regular basis that I'd give them credit on a Sunday dinner. Meaning they could get their food on Sunday and pay me later in the week when they got paid. Or when their check came. Or when they had the money.

And yes, it was okay for a while.

Mrs. Bridges would get her Sunday dinner on credit. Pay me Wednesday.

Mr. Grant would get his Sunday dinner on credit. Pay me Friday.

It worked. People were honest. People paid me back.

But then even that had its faults and turns. That's right. Like I said before, nothing good lasts forever.

The credit system broke down. Yes sir. Because some people will tell a lie for no reason at all, especially for some of their friends. Just to get over on you.

Like if one of the neighbors had a friend from out of the neighborhood come to visit them that day I was giving credit for the Sunday dinners. The regular neighbor would say, "Hey, give my friend a plate of food also on credit."

Or "Give my homeboy a plate on credit."

Or "Give my cousin a plate on credit."

And it would be like three or four of these friends or cousins I'd never seen before. People I didn't know. People who didn't live in the neighborhood. People who had no reason to come back and pay me.

So as you know, yes, I took a chance. And got messed around. And took losses.

Some people never paid me back. Some people disappeared. Some people would see me on the street and cross to the other side to avoid me. That was funny. Like I'm going to beat you up or kill you if you don't pay me for a plate of food I've given you on credit. Please, I do this anyway. The nerve of some people.

So after so many times, of course I stopped.

I had to. I was losing money. I was losing time. I was losing my patience.

These people who started doing this messed it up for the others who really needed something like this in that neighborhood. Because the stores in that neighborhood weren't giving out no credit to no one. You try to buy food on credit at the corner store? They'd laugh you out the door.

Business was very slow in that neighborhood. Money was tight. Jobs were scarce. People were struggling.

So yeah, lots of businesses didn't last long, including small-time hustles like what I was doing. The honest people who really needed this type of hospitality in the neighborhood were very upset and disappointed.

They'd come to me. "Johnny, why'd you stop the credit?"

I'd say, "Because people were taking advantage. I'm sorry. I wish I could keep doing it. But I can't lose money like that. I myself still got to pay rent where I live."

And they understood. But they were still disappointed. And I was disappointed too.

So after a while, I managed to save a little to move out from that neighborhood.

Even though I stopped the credit system there, my reputation was spreading all over the town of Paterson, New Jersey. People were talking.

"You know that guy Johnny who cooks out of his house? Man, his food is good. I heard a lot of people used to buy from him."

"You ever been to Johnny's spot? Get the fish and grits. You'll thank me later. He puts his heart in his food when he cooks it."

"Johnny's oxtails better than any restaurant in town that I know so far I've been to lately."

So once I moved from that neighborhood, I moved to 97 Cedar Street and Summer, Paterson, New Jersey.

And there I had a front window on the first-floor apartment. A big window facing the street. Perfect for doing business.

And I first got to know that neighborhood. And I saw that it was not too different from the neighborhood I just moved from. Run-down buildings. Struggling families. People trying to make it day by day.

But also good people. Hardworking people. People who appreciated good food and fair prices.

So I knew some of the people in the neighborhood. And I talked to them about what I was going to do on the weekends.

I said, "Listen, I'm going to be cooking breakfast and dinner out of my window on Saturdays and Sundays. Spread the word."

And spread the word they did.

And I even made flyers. I went to Staples. Used their copy machine. Designed a simple flyer explaining the type of food and prices and times and days only.

"Fish and Grits, Oxtails and Rice, Saturday and Sunday 7 AM to 2 PM. 97 Cedar Street, First Floor Window."

I printed a hundred copies. Posted them in barbershops and hair salons. Handed them out on the street. Slipped them on cars and homes.

I always got up at 4 AM in the morning. My alarm would go off. Still dark outside. Still quiet.

And I'd get up. No matter how much my legs hurt. No matter how tired I was. No matter how bad the lupus was acting that day.

I'd get up. Because people were counting on me.

And I'd prep the food. Cleaning, preparing everything I'd be cooking in an orderly fashion. Everything had to be ready before 7 AM. And that's a fact. Because they'd be waiting. If I was a couple minutes late, they'd be knocking at my window thinking something was wrong.

I'd open for business about 7 AM in the morning.

And people were already waiting outside the window. Already lined up. Already ready to get that fresh weekend breakfast. Already with their money in their hands. Yes, I loved it.

"Johnny! You open yet?"

"What you got today?"

"Let me get some of the fish and grits!"

So I was always cooking Southern food for them because it was mostly a Southern neighborhood. I used to start with breakfast. Because it was a weekend, most people in that particular neighborhood liked Southern foods.

So I was starting breakfast with some fish and grits. Ham and eggs. Fried chicken and pancakes.

Yes, I kept it simple enough so I could handle it. Knowing I was the only cook. I couldn't do twenty different breakfast options. I couldn't do a big variety of different dishes to choose from like a real restaurant. I had to keep it simple and fast.

And for lunch, it would be hamburgers and hot dogs. Simple. Quick. Easy.

And for dinners, it would be oxtails or turkey wings or baked jerk chicken with a side of vegetables and rice. Or baked mac and cheese. Or candied yams.

It became so popular. And some people really enjoyed it.

It was fun to see people lined up in front of my window. Just waiting for me to start selling breakfast and dinners. And hearing them talk about how good it is.

"Man, this is the best fish and grits I've ever had in a very long time. And that's because most soul food spots in Paterson closed down."

"Johnny, you need to open a restaurant."

I used to say I'd love to but I'm still dealing with some health issues.

"My grandmother used to make oxtails like this. You cooking with love, I can taste it."

There were people from Virginia who got a taste of my fish and grits. Some family members that came to visit on weekend breakfast times. They fell in love with the fish and grits so much that they came every other weekend from the state of Virginia just to get my fish and grits.

Every other weekend. That's a four-hour drive each way. Eight hours round trip. Just for fish and grits.

That's when I knew I had something special.

And it was a time when I wasn't doing it that weekend. Maybe I was too tired. Maybe my lupus was acting up too bad. Maybe I just needed a break.

And they showed up anyway. They would knock on my window. Beg me.

Saying, "Please, can you just serve us the fish and grits? We drove all the way from Virginia just for this. We're not staying up here in the state of Paterson, New Jersey. We just came for the food and a little clothes shopping."

And so they even said, "And could you do a tray to feed twenty people?"

A whole tray. For their family back in Virginia. Yes, that was about a quick two hundred dollars.

So yes, I did it. Even though I was tired. Even though I said I wasn't cooking that weekend. Even though my legs were swollen and my body was aching.

I did it. Because that's two hundred dollars. Because they drove four hours. Because they believed in my food that much.

My fish and grits and oxtails and rice were very popular weekend specials for a lot of people in that neighborhood. No contest. People went crazy for it.

I'd make thirty orders of fish and grits and sell out by 9 AM.

And oxtails and rice with red beans was my most popular dinner also. Those oxtails? Tender. Falling off the bone. Seasoned perfect. Smothered in gravy.

People would be like, "Give me four of them dinners, please."

People would order two plates. One to eat now. One to save for later.

And my prices were definitely affordable but firm. And no one really complained about my prices, so that was a plus in my book.

No matter what type of breakfast or dinners. Fish and grits? Ham and eggs? Fried chicken and pancakes? Oxtails? Turkey wings? Jerk chicken? People were going crazy having a good time eating good food for cheap. Please.

Simple. Fair. No confusion.

But people still tried to negotiate.

"Come on, Johnny, can you do this for me, please?"

I'd be like, "Dammit." It never fails. Someone always got to start it.

"Johnny, I only got this much, can you give me a dinner anyway?"

"Johnny, I'm a regular, can't you give me a discount?"

Or try to complain.

"This portion is smaller than last time."

"Why you only giving me three pieces of oxtail?"

"My cousin said you gave him more rice than this."

Or try to get over on me.

And because I didn't let them have their way on getting over on me, yes, of course they gave me some type of problems.

Either they would curse me out.

"F you, Johnny! Your food ain't even that good!"

"You think you're special because you can cook? Man, get out of here with that!"

Or try to turn the neighbors against me. Going around the neighborhood. Talking trash. Or try to stop neighbors from buying from me. By telling people the food is not good and not fresh.

"Don't buy from Johnny. I heard his sister cooks most of the food anyway."

"I heard he don't look out for people who spend good money with him."

"I heard he got a chip on his shoulder if you don't tip him."

None of it was true. All of it was lies. But lies spread fast in a small neighborhood.

And there were more lies. That I lived in a house where a lot of guys hustle drugs out of it. That my apartment was dirty. My apartment was clean. I kept everything sanitized. I took pride in my cooking space. And trust me, I definitely wouldn't try to live right in the mix of drug dealers.

But people say what they want to say when they're mad they didn't get their way.

So slowly I started to slow down on the number of meals I cooked on a weekend. I wasn't making many meals during the week. Just on weekends.

And I was making about thirty breakfasts and thirty dinners. So that's both days, Saturday and Sunday. So about sixty meals a week. Thirty breakfasts, thirty dinners, that's it.

And that was about 240 meals a month. Just on the weekend. That's still really a lot. Plus I was starting my other side hustles I was coming up with.

So I stopped once it started getting out of control.

For one, my electric and gas was almost half of what I was paying for rent. My rent was one price and my electric was another. It started taking a toll on me.

Because I was cooking all day Saturday. All day Sunday. Oven on. Stove on. Everything running hot. The bills were eating up my profits.

It started to be overwhelming.

My legs started getting too bad with the varicose veins. All that standing. All that moving around the kitchen. All that cooking. My legs would swell up so big I couldn't get my shoes on.

My lupus started being very active. The stress. The lack of sleep. The physical strain. All of it was triggering flare-ups. And of course, people didn't care because it's not them having to deal with that type of health issues.

I was trying to do something good for the community. I was selling good food at fair prices. I was feeding people who couldn't afford restaurants. I was giving people a reason to stay in the neighborhood instead of leaving.

But instead of appreciating it, some people tried to take advantage.

And on top of it, my landlord said he didn't like the traffic. Of course, that was coming sooner or later.

He came to me one day. "Johnny, I got neighbors complaining about all the people coming to your window. This is a residential building. Not a restaurant."

Or the fact I got a weekend business going on his properties.

"You need a business license for this. You need permits. You need insurance. I can't have you running a restaurant out of my building."

And the next-door neighbors that were living in the same residential facility I was living in didn't like the idea either.

"It smells like food all the time."

"People are too loud in the morning."

"There's trash everywhere from all your customers."

And the phone calls just never stopped. People were calling my phone all hours of the night.

2 AM. "Johnny, you cooking tomorrow?"

4 AM. "Johnny, can you make me a special order?"

6 AM. "Johnny, you up yet? When you opening?"

People would come knock on my window all hours of the morning and night. Before I even opened. After I already closed.

Knock knock knock. "Johnny! You in there?"

Knock knock knock. "Johnny! I know you got food left!"

And wouldn't take no for an answer.

"Come on, Johnny, just one plate."

"Johnny, please, I'm hungry."

"Johnny, I got money, I'll pay you extra."

I actually had to move out of the neighborhood. Because then they started to be disrespectful by not stopping calling my phone or knocking on my window. Even after I told them I was done. Even after I said no more. They kept coming. Kept calling. Kept demanding. To where I had to change my phone number and after a while I had to move from the area. That's how out of control people were getting.

And why I had to stop also because my health was getting worse. So I said to myself, either my health or my business. I went with my health.

So I stopped it.

I told people in the neighborhood, "I am not doing it no more. I'm sorry. I want to get another hustle going on."

Because I couldn't get any sleep or rest on weekends or weekdays. I was exhausted. I was in pain. I was watching my health deteriorate.

And I was always in search to find a hustle to meet my situation of living with lupus. Something that wouldn't be a strain on my legs and the lupus.

But this? This wasn't it. This was destroying my health while I was trying to help my community.

I was making money, yes. But I was losing my body. I was losing my peace. I was losing myself.

And no amount of money is worth that.

So I stopped. I moved. I started over somewhere else.

But the lessons stayed with me. The reputation stayed with me. The knowledge that I could cook food that people would drive four hours to get. That stayed with me too.

And that's what kept me going. Knowing that someday, when my health was better, when I had the right setup, when I had the proper support, I could do it again.

The right way. The sustainable way. The way that feeds the community without destroying the cook in the process.

Chapter 9
How I Ignore the Negativity to Keep A Positive Mindset

So as I started trying different gigs to earn money, I had people telling me it was stupid. Saying it's a bad idea. Or even saying I'm playing myself out. I'm degrading myself.

People were saying all kinds of negative things about my hustle. About my ideas. About what I was doing to survive.

I can remember this one guy by the name of Mr. T.J. Reese. Oh yes, the fake friend who laughed behind my back and was lying to my face. Saying, "Yeah, that's a cool idea." And once I turned my back, he was laughing and talking down on me and my ideas.

So like I said before, as I was coming up with these ideas to support myself, I remember there was this guy who I thought was a cool alright homeboy. His name was T.J. Reese.

Man, oh man, he surprised me with his charm. He acted like he liked my ideas of quick hustles I was coming up with. Every time he'd see me, he'd stop by. Act all interested.

"Hey Johnny, what you got going on today? What's the new hustle?"

And I'd tell him. Because I thought he was cool, an okay dude. I thought he was in my corner. I thought he was supporting me in some sort of way. Surprise, surprise how people really can disguise themselves to act like they're cool but on the real, they're nothing but a fool.

I kind of knew something wasn't right about this dude T.J. Reese. The simple fact is all you ever did was ask me about my business but never was supporting my business I had going on at the time.

But God always watches over His anointed child. See how God ended up letting me meet this honest fellow by the name of Mr. Phillips. He pulled me to the side one day and told me something I needed to hear.

He said, "Please, Johnny, you are a cool dude. I have nothing against you. And I see your struggles. Your positive ideas are good. It's better than doing something illegal. I'd take your ideas any day. Trust me, my brother. But do me a favor. Please stop telling everyone your ideas. Because people who you think are for you really are not. They are against you. They don't want to see you win. And they're stealing your ideas."

I said, "Yeah? So what made you say all this to me, Mr. Phillips? Because the minute that guy T.J. Reese finds out about your new ideas and hustles, he starts talking trash about you, brother."

So I said, "What did you hear T.J. Reese say about me?"

So Mr. Phillips said, "Well, I'll tell you. T.J. Reese tells everyone you're living in a fantasy world with all your stupid ideas."

So I said, "Word up? What type of other things was he saying, Mr. Phillips?"

He said, "That you were crazy. And you are going to make a fool out of yourself trying to think you're going to pull off your side hustles to make ends meet."

"He said, 'Nobody is going to support nobody's home-made food from out of his house.'"

"'Nobody is not going to let him cut their hair out in their backyard!'"

"'Who does he think he is trying to do all these side hustles in the streets like this?'"

So Mr. Phillips said he told him, "Hey, it's positive. I'm for it. Everything is worth a try."

And Mr. T.J. Reese told Mr. Phillips, "You know what? You're crazy also. I knew I shouldn't have told you how I feel about Johnny's hustles."

So the next time I saw T.J. Reese, I started thinking about what Mr. Phillips said. You know, about T.J. Reese, that he was laughing behind my back about all my side hustles I got going on.

So he tried to have a conversation like we usually do when he stops through my area.

And I told him, "Pardon me, Mr. T.J. Reese, but I got a hustle I got to keep going. I don't have time to talk too much. Especially to backstabbing phony old men who are supposed to be a minister of a church. Please go back and do your homework. Especially with God. Because even you still got lots to learn about being a positive, God-given human being."

And I walked away.

I didn't argue. I didn't curse him out. I didn't get mad.

I just let him know I knew. And I kept it moving.

So I thank God for the people who were in my corner who would come back to me. Telling me everything that was being said. So that I can stay on point of my surroundings.

And yes, I definitely appreciated that. Because at least I knew who was real and who wasn't.

So as I gave the ideas a try, some took off and some didn't. Yes, that's the way life works out with things, you know.

But the ones that took off made up for the ones that didn't.

I mean, I started making money to pay bills. Like my electric and gas company. And to take transportation to where I needed to go.

So my driver's license was suspended because of letting close friends drive my car and getting tickets in my name, and they were not telling me. So as time went on, the tickets were piling up.

From parking tickets from not moving the car when it's street cleaning. Not stopping at stop signs. And not using turning signals when making a turn.

The tickets came up to a lot of money I didn't have or have saved up. The tickets came up to $2,000.

That was way out of my league at that time in life. So I had to let my license get suspended.

And as time went on, the fine went up.

So I was stuck on: How am I going to get my license back? And how am I going to pay these fines for all these tickets?

Seventeen years without a license. I can't live like this. My driver's license is my life right about now. I've been without a license for seventeen years.

Think about that. That's almost two decades.

Seventeen years of walking everywhere. Seventeen years of catching buses. Seventeen years of asking people for rides. Seventeen years of carrying grocery bags on my feet. Seventeen years of my legs swelling because I had to walk so much.

Seventeen years of depending on other people just to get around.

Just had to find a way to get my license back. To get my license back is like being born again.

So I actually got up enough money to restore my driver's license with all the side hustles I had going on at the time.

But after a long seventeen years of getting my license back, I tell you, it felt so good. It almost felt like I was born all over again. It felt like I hit the Mega Millions. It felt like I had a brand new life.

Because all I could think of was: Wow, now I can give my legs a break and make better moves with myself.

I can take myself to the doctors and don't have to ask anybody.

I can take myself to better supermarkets and don't have to settle for these high-price, low-budget, bad food side markets in my community.

I can finally get a break from doing a lot of walking long distance. Struggling with eight shopping bags walking up the streets.

That license meant freedom. That license meant independence. That license meant I didn't have to depend on people who might talk behind my back.

And yes, I still had more ideas I wanted to give a try, like this new idea that I wanted to start. Renting out my car. It seemed to sound like a good idea at the time. I figured everyone was looking for an affordable car rental to do all their running around, to take care of their important business. I figured why not.

I had given so many ideas a try. And they mostly worked for me. But nope, this idea definitely failed me.

So I just had to slow it down and give it a break because of my legs. And when the weather got too hot or too cold, my lupus would act up.

But this one idea I had didn't go well. It failed.

I remember buying a used car for $700. I knew a little mechanical work. I did it. Got the car to drive from A to C. That means it would get you to do some local area only driving. Like from my home to downtown area. That's like twenty to thirty blocks.

I tried renting out the car to neighbors to do their grocery shopping. Or go run around to do some errands for themselves.

I put my trust into them on the fact they lived next door. Same block. And we see each other every day. And they had a family and a job.

But all people are not responsible.

So I guess you know I almost got back in the same position of getting my license suspended.

One of the neighbors who rented the car got a ticket. Didn't tell no one.

I found out in time. I paid it. The ticket was $50.

Thank God I had enough money on hand to pay that quickly.

So I had to think: Was that a sign of not starting that type of business? Especially when you're having someone using a car within your name.

So that idea of a hustle didn't go well. It failed.

I definitely had to learn my lesson from the last time with this one. I have to always keep in mind that trust does have its limits.

What did I learn from that failed idea? I tell you.

I learned that even good people make mistakes. Even responsible people get tickets. Even neighbors you see every day can mess up your situation without meaning to.

I learned that some hustles look good on paper but don't work in real life.

I learned that putting your name on anything, whether it's a car or a lease or a loan, is a risk. And when you got lupus and you're barely surviving, you can't afford risks like that.

I learned to be more careful. More selective. More protective of the little bit I had going on at the time.

Because one $50 ticket could have turned into a suspended license again. And I couldn't go back to that. Not after seventeen years.

So yeah, I stayed praying for protection and discernment.

So as time went on, as I sat back in my house and prayed to God:

"Please lead me in the right directions in life."

"Please keep me away from people who will try to hurt me in some type of manner."

"Please, God, let me recognize certain people who are up to no good."

"Please let me stay aware of not just letting people in my life who are using me and taking advantage of me and my situation."

"Taking my kindness for granted. Or because I'm suffering with lupus and I'll need some help at some time."

"Because even though I do need help every now and then, God, I always want people to know it's my lupus, my problem."

"Not ever trying to put it off on nobody or no one."

"This is definitely one of the reasons for writing this book."

And so, as I started moving on with myself, with many ideas I was trying to get going to support myself with living arrangements, some associates who I used to deal with noticed I was not being bothered anymore with too many people from my past.

So one of these guys from my past finally came around one day and asked, "Can he talk to me?"

And the talk was about an apology.

He told me he was sorry about what he said about my ideas. "And I never knew about your health situation and that you were suffering from lupus."

I said, "Mr. T.J. Reese, let me tell you first: I'll appreciate the fact you are apologizing. I accept."

"But I don't be going around telling people I have lupus. Because it's not their problem."

"Lupus is my problem. God blessed me with lupus. And we are both doing alright with not spreading the news about our problems we go through."

"Thank you."

And I moved on.

And so I am always being careful now on how I can recognize genuine people. Just to stay away from the negative people.

As time went on, God helped me recognize genuine people versus negative people. Also especially the ones who give off negative energy. And how I knew this person was genuine. Because one of the genuine reasons was this person always supported everything that was positive I did as a business. And never asked for any favors that would cost me or cause me any harm.

I recognize negative energy the first time I meet someone.

And right away, they start to tell me:

"I don't think that's a good idea."

"I did that before. It didn't work out."

"Can I borrow some money?"

"Can I get a ride somewhere?"

Basically, what I am saying is: this person or persons don't even know me that well. And already they're begging and asking me for everything.

So I keep it moving away from these types of individuals. So that I can keep a safe mindset and stay from getting corrupted by these negative individuals.

And here's how I tell the difference:

Genuine concern sounds like: "Johnny, I support what you're doing, but have you thought about this problem? Let me help you figure it out."

Negative energy sounds like: "That's stupid. Nobody's going to buy that. You're wasting your time."

Genuine people offer solutions. Negative people offer criticism.

Genuine people ask how they can help. Negative people ask what you can do for them.

Genuine people celebrate when you win. Negative people get quiet or make excuses.

Genuine people stick around when things are hard. Negative people disappear and come back when things are good.

That's how I know. That's how God showed me.

And I try to stay on this type of level and attitude to keep me aware, for one. And to keep me from thinking about negative thoughts about someone also.

And when I do think negative thoughts about anyone, I sit back and check within myself.

Saying to myself: "Hold up, Johnny. You know how life is with a lot of things in life. So just slow down. Ask God to forgive you for almost thinking negative about someone."

"No one is perfect. So brush it off and keep on your journey. Because only you know the bigger picture you're working on."

Because sometimes the negative thoughts come from me. Not from other people.

Sometimes I'm the one doubting myself. Sometimes I'm the one saying, "This won't work. You can't do this. You're too sick. Your legs are too bad."

And when those thoughts come, I have to stop. I have to pray. I have to remind myself:

God didn't bring me this far to leave me.

God didn't give me lupus to destroy me. He gave it to me to teach me.

God didn't put these ideas in my head for them to fail. He put them there for me to try.

So I brush off the negative thoughts. I play my music. I pray. And I keep going.

And so let me also tell you about the two to three people I can always count on.

So I am always thinking of the two to three people who I can count on when things are tough. Or when I need to talk to someone or a shoulder to lean on.

My fiancée.

And two old family members that always guided me in the right path.

These are the people who never doubted me. Never laughed behind my back. Never told me my ideas were stupid.

These are the people who saw me at my worst and still believed in me.

These are the people who know about my lupus and never made me feel like a burden.

These are the people who, when I call them at 2 AM because the pain is too bad and I can't sleep, they answer the phone.

These are my people. My real people.

And I thank God for them every single day.

So yes, I always got to keep my protective shield so I can stay negative proof and sucker free.

And once I did that, I knew none of those negative people can say anything that was negative that can get in my way.

Because as you know, like I said before, once I start to play my favorite music by Earth, Wind & Fire, "Keep Your Head to the Sky," well, I did.

And I also kept my mind on my money and goals. To reaching my goals.

And that's how I got to stay focused.

And to building a protective shield that was negative proof and sucker free from all who were negative against me.

Here's how I built that shield:

First: I stopped sharing my ideas with everyone. Only the real ones get to know what I'm working on.

Second: I stopped arguing with people who doubt me. Let them talk. Let them laugh. I'll show them with results.

Third: I surrounded myself with my two to three real people. Quality over quantity.

Fourth: I prayed every day for discernment. For God to show me who's real and who's fake.

Fifth: I played my music. Earth, Wind & Fire. "Keep Your Head to the Sky." That music is my armor.

Sixth: I kept my eyes on my goals. Not on the haters. Not on the doubters. On my goals.

Seventh: I forgave people like T.J. Reese. Not for them. For me. Because holding onto anger is heavy. And I got enough to carry with lupus.

That's my shield. That's how I stay protected. That's how I keep negativity from stopping my progress.

Yes, because the proof is in the results that I accomplished throughout my journey.

All those people who said my ideas were stupid? I made money anyway.

All those people who said nobody would buy my food? I had people driving from Virginia for my fish and grits.

All those people who said I was degrading myself cutting hair in backyards? I made enough money to get my license back after seventeen years.

All those people who laughed behind my back? They're still in the same place doing the same things. And I'm still moving forward.

So let them talk. Let them laugh. Let them doubt.

I'll keep my head to the sky. I'll keep my faith in God. I'll keep my focus on my goals.

Because at the end of the day, it's my lupus, my problem. And I'm handling it my way.

And nobody's negativity can stop what God has planned for me.

Chapter 10
How I Had to Learn to Have Patience With All Things in My Life

Well, as you know, everything doesn't happen overnight. Especially good things. Most of anything and everything that will be a blessing, that will be a good positive impact on your life, to improve it, to make it easier so you can live comfortably, has its challenging situations.

So a lot of times I just wanted to give up on all my ideas and projects I was working on. Because most of the times it seemed to be taking too long for me to get off the ground. So I had to think hard, pray hard, and more just to come up with: How can I train myself to have patience on all these projects I am working on?

So as I used to cook breakfast and dinners, I started meditating and focusing on my cooking. And I started saying to myself, "Well, I guess I can use the same patience strategy, same remedies I use when I cook my breakfast and dinners. Using the same method for my ideas and projects."

Because when you're cooking, you can't rush. You can't turn the heat up too high or you'll burn the food. You can't pull the chicken out the oven before it's done or you'll make people sick. You have to let it cook. You have to wait. You have to trust the process.

And that's how I started to develop discipline for myself. Of having patience for the positive movements in my life.

So once I started having patience, it started paying off for me. And as time went by, it started getting a little easier to deal with the time and effort. Especially once it started paying off. Again and again. I saw that most of my ideas were coming to light. My vision of the ideas was clearer. My mind seemed less cluttered.

I even made a schedule on how much time each day was put to the side to where I would spend working on each idea. And every hour, to every day, to every week, to every month, I got closer to completing most of my ideas and projects I was working on for so long.

I started making this "having patience" as a daily routine. And a mandatory part of my life and style I lived by. I took an oath and made a promise to myself: I will learn how to control myself with having patience. And I won't let negative things and people who are around me while on my journey distract me or take me off my focus of what I am working on. That's going to upgrade my life and make me a better me for this time and this future.

I can remember the longest project I ever worked on was house cleanups.

I saved up about $600 and bought myself a junk cargo van. Used. From a private owner who wasn't using it anymore because he had too many other vehicles. So I got lucky and he gave it to me really cheap. But it needed repairs: a new battery, oil change, and two new tires.

Once I purchased the vehicle, I couldn't drive it right away because of the repairs it needed. I had to let the guy who I purchased it from hold the vehicle until I got the paperwork together on it. And then save up a little more money for the repairs it needed.

And so once that was done, I sat back in my house to do some thinking on how am I going to put this business plan together. And stick with it. Because I am tired of keep switching hustles and different ways of making money to help support myself.

So I got my planning pad and started writing everything down about how I would write down everything I will need and do. And I would keep this pad on me everywhere I go. Taking down notes from everything that would pop up or come to my mind.

I first purchased cleaning supplies and garbage bags. Things like brooms and shovels, towels, Ajax and bleach, and other cleaning tools.

Then I started to pass the word around the neighborhood that I do small apartment and house cleanups. So they said, "What do you mean?"

I said, "I will clean up any room in the house that you don't want to be bothered with because it's too much for you."

"What type of cleaning?"

"I'll sweep, mop, or vacuum. I'll spray and wipe down walls and dust off the furniture in that room only. How much I charge per room is $30."

So I kept this side hustle project going on for six months. It got popular. My clientele got up.

So yes, I definitely decided to hire some help. I got two close friends to help me. One named Mr. Tapiary Justin and the other named Ford Brassing.

So the two of them played a part of this side hustle by putting in the garbage in the bags and sweeping and mopping the floors. I'd do the dusting and spraying down the walls.

We made a decent amount of money throughout the weekly basis. Most neighbors heard about how good we were. And when they did business with us, they wanted the whole three-to-four-bedroom apartment done.

So we got about three to four apartments a week. Grossing about 480 a week. Giving my two coworkers 130 apiece. And the rest of the money I'd put back into cleaning supplies and the maintenance work on the vehicle.

I didn't care about me bringing home a lot of money at that time. As long as the two friends that worked for me were satisfied with their pay. Plus, they kept all the tips. Of course, they ate free most of the time because I still was cooking food to feed five to six people. So I always offered them some before we started to work.

And why I had to slow down on this hustle a little bit is once my lupus got too active. Because the business had me going nonstop with a steady flow. My lupus, I guess, got upset because I wasn't taking no breaks to rest myself and letting my body cooperate from working every day. Yes, that's the way lupus works. You don't rest, your lupus doesn't rest either. That's the way of lupus telling you to play fair. I take it easy on you while you trying to maintain a decent lifestyle, you return a favor and take it easy on me. Remember, I am still here for life. You can't get rid of lupus, just treatment. And I suggest you treat lupus with respect. When the body says rest, rest, just as simple as that.

So business was good for a little while. Like a year and a half. My lupus just was getting too active. I had to slow it down.

This is what's been happening to me most of my life so far since I've been dealing with lupus. I've always got to catch it when I notice the lupus starts to be so active.

Like my face will flare up. My body will start to ache with arthritis. My fingers, wrists, and hands. Including shoulders and arms. So before it gets too bad that I can't do for myself, I slow it down. Take it easy until I can get my lupus back on track.

I remember there were so many times I wanted to give up on a project.

But I started to think about where I came from. When I had no car. No money at all. Or no one I could call on for any help.

So this is why I'm always thankful for having God in my life to help me find that strength in my mind. So I can have a strong mind to have the willpower of faith to keep moving on with my life. So I can see one of the projects I started actually get finished for once in my life.

So that's when I stopped and said to myself, "Why am I rushing? Who am I racing against?"

So as I still try to keep my life going and projects I am trying to figure out, goals I am trying to accomplish, I'll say it again and again:

"Why am I rushing everything? Who am I racing against? Someone or time?"

"I don't rush when I am cooking. I don't rush when I put together a meal that will be a state of art. So let me try the same thing with what I am trying to do with my life and projects I am working on."

And I did just that. And I found myself less stressed and less confused about when and where I am going to start a new project.

And as I continue to do my daily schedule, I'll start at one time and be finished at another time. My daily schedule looks okay. But we know it can be better if we were to reach our goals in life sooner than we can.

So every day is about the same for me. Only thing different is the time. Reasons why I am saying this: because I do almost the same routine for myself to keep me going for the projects I am working on.

I get up around 4 AM. Take my shower and my meds with my smoothie. I sit back, relax for about a half hour until my body feels comfortable to start moving.

I get up and do a daily stretch. Exercise bike. Punch the heavy bag. And do wall pushups and dips. That's when you lean up against the wall and push yourself up and away from it. Same with the dips. And I do a few squats. About 100 every other day. Sometimes every day. Depends on how I feel.

I do a couple of dumbbell curls with 10 pounds and 20 pounds. I relax for thirty minutes after the workout and then start my day.

So all the workout and getting ready for my day, it takes me two hours, sometimes three, before I leave out the house. Because most of the time I'll take my dinner for the night and prep it first after working out.

So when I go out to do my running around, because that most of the times takes another three to four hours. So yes, I do two to three hours getting ready to three hours of running around taking care of business. So yes, my day is very busy of taking care of myself and my home.

Some projects I had to delay. Like the clothing line and magazine.

Some projects I was working on in the past took too long to where I had to delay it and put it on hold. That project was my own clothing line and my own magazine.

My clothing was called R.S.P. Stands for Realistic Super Products. And the name of the magazine company was called Let's Get Together.

See, the reasons for the clothing line is to let people know they are buying top quality products. And it will be super strong to last you because it is made out of the best products.

And the reasons for the magazine company came about: How people in my position were, where they can't work because of a disability of a health issue. Also, people who were on drugs and trying to get their lives back in order and on the right track. This is why the magazine is called Let's Get Together.

The reasons why I had to delay these two projects is because of getting people to model for the clothing line. Because of not being paid the money they wanted. I offered $25 to just take pictures with a T-shirt representing the name of the clothing line. They wanted $100.

So I had to put that on hold.

I put the magazine on hold because it was hard to get people to tell their story to me and take their pictures to put in the magazine.

So yes, I definitely had a couple of projects I had to delay.

But I did get to do the two projects. And it lasted for the summer only. I managed to get four people to model off my T-shirts. And I got two people to tell a little story about themselves trying to get their life back together again. But I never got to print it in a magazine.

And let me tell you how lupus taught me patience I never had before.

If you experience the pain and suffering lupus can bring to your body, to your life, just having the mindset to even bear the tricks of it punishing different body parts of your body, oh, trust me, you will learn how to have patience. And I mean lots of patience. Trust me.

Because when lupus is active, you can't rush anything. You can't force your body to do what it won't do. You can't speed up healing. You can't make the pain stop on your schedule.

You have to wait. You have to let your body rest. You have to give the medication time to work. You have to trust that the flare will pass eventually.

That's patience you can't learn from a book. That's patience you earn through suffering.

And so what techniques do I use when I don't have patience and I am frustrated?

I cut my day in half by doing a half workout and eating small breakfast and dinners for that day. And I won't spend too much time doing any running around. Because that also takes a lot out of me and my little pocket change and gas for my car.

I pray. I sit still. I play my music. I remind myself that everything I've accomplished so far came from waiting. From not giving up. From trusting God's timing instead of my own.

And let me tell you what good came from waiting. Everything that I didn't expect.

So I am so glad I learned how to wait for certain things I wanted to do. I waited for certain things I wanted in life.

Like when I used to start different projects, I waited to see what this person was about before including him into my projects. So that saved me some money and kept me away from problems.

I'm glad I waited to buy a car. Because around New Years' time, a lot of vehicles I was looking for were very cheap.

When I was looking for clothing for different occasions and it had to be a special type of occasion like a wedding, I got myself a two-piece men's suit at a discount because I waited.

I remember when I was waiting for a certain Broadway show to come out and tickets were too expensive. I waited and caught them on sale for that year of the season.

Yes, of course, I got so much good out of waiting. It became part of my therapy in life.

Well, let me start by saying: How do I balance patience for my bills? Ha ha, I had no choice but to learn to have patience on that occasion.

Why? Well, because if you're living with a health issue that can keep you from being steady with working or trying to make money on the side, if that don't teach you, I don't know what will.

That is like a number one thing someone with only treatable health issues will learn: to have patience. Especially if you're not well off financially. And you don't have a family that cares to help you or care for your well-being.

If you're not born into money. If you don't have reliable family or friends, whoever you have been dealing with from your past to present to future, you are going to be in big disappointments in life if you don't practice patience with yourself.

And if you don't want to be disciplined with yourself on a patience level, all you will do is suffer. And you will be putting yourself in that position. Because you should know better. You knew nobody was going to help you out. You knew nobody was just going to give you money, especially to pay your bills. What about their bills? LOL.

Things change. People are always changing quicker than things. So act like you know. If you never want to be in that position, please, I tell you, practice patience.

I wish I knew what I know now when I was in my teenage years. Because I was in a position to be set really financially right with myself.

I say this by saying: I was involved with so much work. Well connected with people who were in position to hire me for everything at their place of employment.

I was involved with sports and modeling. I was working two to three jobs all my teen years from 14 years of age. I worked at IHOP and for the city. And summertime at a youth camp.

So yes, I would tell myself: Start learning how to have patience because you will need it in the long run. Trust me, the world will get very hard for a person like you living with health issues. And you can't expect no one to be there for you. Because no one owes you anything.

Save your money. Don't spend it all on clothes and shoes and trying to impress people. Put some away. Even if it's just $20 a paycheck. Start building.

Be patient with people. Not everyone is going to move at your speed. Not everyone is going to understand your vision. Not everyone is going to support you. And that's okay. Keep moving.

But have patience with yourself. You're going to make mistakes. You're going to fail at some things. You're going to have setbacks. That's part of the journey. Don't beat yourself up. Learn and keep going.

And most importantly: Be patient with God. He's got a plan. Even when you can't see it. Even when it doesn't make sense. Even when lupus is kicking your ass and you're wondering why this is happening to you. Trust His timing. Not yours.

Because everything I have now, everything I've built, everything I've learned, came from waiting. Came from not giving up when things were taking too long. Came from trusting the process even when I wanted to quit.

That's what patience gave me. That's what it will give you too.

Chapter 11
Mastering the Craft I Love
Most in Life

If you are an artist or know anything about art, it only comes out eye-catching and starts to say something to the people who admire it or find it interesting. And yes, you will be hypnotized and stuck in the moment of time wondering how amazing, how beautiful this artwork is.

You yourself would want to meet the artist who created this unique design or beautiful picture. Just to ask: What were you thinking at the time you were doing this artwork? What were you feeling? What were you trying to say?

Yes, art can be a powerful meditating therapy session for the mind, the heart, also the soul of a human or animal.

Yes, I am quite sure by now you all know that animals are fascinated by pretty artworks. They stop. They stare. They tilt their heads. Something in the colors or shapes speaks to them too.

I remember being in fifth grade. And I ended up doing an incredible Hulk drawing that made me a superstar. It was a sketch of the Incredible Hulk.

I was in the fifth grade. And it was an art contest going on among the students. It was about four different classes that were participating. Four students from each classroom. And I won first place.

I felt like I was a superstar. I felt like I was on top of the world. Especially when all the students in the school were cheering for me. My artwork was talked about that whole school year.

The name of the school was Number Eleven Elementary Grammar School. That school only goes up to the fifth grade. The school teachers in that school were very nice. They cared so much about the students there.

I can remember one teacher who stood out from the others. She went by the name Ms. Joseph. She was all the students' favorite mom teacher. She looked just like the mom who plays on The Cosby Show. The one they called Claire.

And I can remember my mom's artwork also. It was a picture of an Indian woman who lived in South America.

The way my mom drew was different from mine. I was all about action. Superheroes. Movement. My mom was about faces. About capturing something in a person's eyes. About showing who they were inside, not just what they looked like outside.

I wish I had her artwork still. I don't know what happened to it. Maybe it got lost when we moved. Maybe it got damaged. Maybe someone has it somewhere. But I remember looking at it and thinking: That's what I want to do. I want to make people feel something when they see my work.

From drawing faces to shaping faces is also why I became a barber.

So because I saw how art can have a big impact on a person, on a person's life, I started to learn how to cut hair and create different styles of a desired design of their liking.

It made the person happy. It even made the person have a different type of glow with themselves. It made people also determined to change their lifestyle for the best of themselves.

And when I saw I could do amazing things in people's lives, I decided to go to barber school. Because it was part of art. Still a lot to be learned in the art world. But this time, the canvas was a person's head. The paintbrush was clippers and scissors. The masterpiece was confidence. Self-worth. Hope.

So around twelve years old, I remember my first job at Mac's Ideal Barbershop. But not cutting hair, but sweeping up the hair. To wiping down all the mirrors.

I can remember the first time I cut someone's hair. I also was about twelve years old. The owner of the barbershop I worked for asked me if I want to learn, I will first have to bring one of my friends to practice on. So yes, it all started when I used to hang in front of a barbershop on East 18th and 12th Avenue in Paterson,

New Jersey. The shop was called Mac's Ideal Barbershop.

So one day, as I used to sit outside in front of the barbershop looking inside at the owner of the barbershop cut hair, he came outside and told me: "Hey, you little boy, didn't your parents ever tell you that you should never sit in front of someone's business?"

I thought I was in trouble. I thought he was going to yell at me or chase me away.

Then he told me, "Come inside. Sit down." Then he asked me if I wanted a job. I said, "Yes."

So he said, "Oh no, not cutting hair. But to sweep and mop my floors and clean my mirrors once I am closed."

So I said, "Yeah, I can do that."

So he told me every day to be there in the barbershop at 6 PM. And I did. And I stayed doing that type of work for six months. And he would pay me $2 a day. The work I did only took me 40 minutes to do and finish up.

And then came the day he asked me if I wanted to learn how to cut hair. I said, "Yes, I do."

So he told me to bring one of my friends to the barbershop and I could practice on their hair. And I did. And it went great. He said it was okay for my first time. "But you will have to practice a lot."

So every weekend I'd bring a different friend to the barbershop and cut their hair. And slowly but shortly, I went from okay to good. My friends were my training ground. Some haircuts came out better than others. Some of my friends walked out looking sharp. Some walked out looking like they lost a fight with a lawnmower. But they all let me practice. And that's how I learned.

I can remember the most complicated haircut I ever did was a mid-fade.

That type of haircut looks easy but is very difficult. Especially if you are doing it on a person who has salt and pepper hair. That's a person who has hair with black scattered around the top and bottom and gray hair in between all the black hair.

Because while you're cutting the hair, the gray hair can confuse you. And you will lose yourself in the haircut, of what type of haircut you're doing. The gray blends with the skin in certain lights. You think you're done blending, but you're not. You think the fade is even, but it's not. You have to keep checking from different angles. Keep adjusting. Keep blending. One wrong move and the whole fade is ruined.

So yes, I decided to go to barbering school. And got my license to be a master barber. And the journey that I went through during that process was a wonderful life experience.

The barbering school I attended was hands-on. They had a deal going on with all homeless shelters in NYC to give haircuts to the homeless people for $3.

So I met all walks of lifestyles while giving haircuts to the people of homeless shelters. And finding out what made them give up on life, what stopped them from being successful, or why they just were not wanting to do good in their life. Every person had a story. Every story was different. But the pain was the same. Loss. Addiction. Mental illness. Bad choices. Bad luck. Sometimes a combination of all of it.

So once I completed a haircut on each one, they were amazed. And started to have a change of mind. A change of heart. Didn't want to be in that position in their lives anymore. And just knowing I was the cause of that type of impact, it made me feel really good. Like I was doing more than cutting hair. I was giving people a reason to try again. To believe they were worth something. To look in the mirror and see a person, not a problem.

And I can remember when I helped this homeless man from the shelter in NYC. When the homeless man came into the barber school, he needed someone to cut his hair in an emergency.

So let me begin telling you what had happened. The homeless man was sleeping in the streets before getting into the shelter. So while he was sleeping, some street kids poured crazy glue into his hair. Like big tubes. And they tried to cover his entire head.

He had long hair that hung down to his back. Like Fabio. He was a Caucasian middle-aged man, about fifty-five years of age. His name was Hills.

And when he came into the barber school for someone to help him, because the barbers in the school were all students, they were intimidated to touch him and his hair. They were kind of scared. Like they were going to catch something. Or if they could handle a job like that without hurting him.

So they asked me. And I said, "Yes, I'll do it for him." Because I love a challenge. And I thought about: What if I was in that position? I would want someone to help me.

So I did it. And the man had tears coming out of his eyes. And he just kept telling me, "Thank you," over and over. I said, "It's okay. You will be alright now. I've gotten all the hair that had crazy glue on it."

And yes, I have pictures of the man before and after the haircut. Before, he looked defeated. Humiliated. Like the world had beaten him down and he had nothing left. After, he looked human again. Dignified. Like he mattered. Like he had value.

And so there was another man that was sitting in the barber school waiting for his turn to get a haircut. And he was watching me cut the homeless man's hair that had crazy glue on top.

So he came over to me and asked me to cut his hair. Because he saw that I took my time and I had a lot of patience with the man I just cut.

And he told me, "That is what I'm looking for. Someone to take their time and to please have patience with me. Because this is my first haircut ever in life."

And I showed him that I care about how I feel when cutting someone's hair. He was a Black American professor from one of the colleges in NYC. He was about fifty or sixty years old. And yes, I have pictures before and after the haircut of the man. His name was Mr. Washington.

Think about that. Fifty or sixty years old. Never had a haircut in his life. That's not just about hair. That's about identity. That's about control. That's about finally deciding to let someone close enough to change something about you. And he trusted me to be that person. That's an honor. That's a responsibility I didn't take lightly.

The barber school was a true life lesson taught by some real knowledgeable, skillful teachers. They not only taught me how to cut but also fed me some of their history on how they got started.

They all had an interesting background of themselves. One served time in the military. One was a security guard. One was homeless. And one had a disability.

I took heed to all. But two of them stood out from the rest.

The one from the military, his name is Mr. Dee. He taught me how to never give up. Never think you know it all. And to never stop wanting to learn. It's never enough. New styles of haircutting are being created every day.

Mr. Dee would say, "The minute you think you've mastered barbering, that's the minute you stop growing. And the minute you stop growing, you start dying. Not physically. But professionally. Creatively. You become stagnant. You become irrelevant. So stay hungry. Stay curious. Stay humble."

And that stuck with me. Not just in barbering. But in life. Never stop learning. Never stop growing. Never stop pushing yourself to be better than you were yesterday.

And the one with a disability. For the record, let me explain. No, he's not mute or special educated. He was blessed by God with one arm that works and one arm that didn't function.

So people of the world named him the One Arm Barber. He's real. You can look him up anywhere. Because he cut hair all over NYC five boroughs. He also appeared on the news several times and was named number one barber in New York State.

He taught me how to control the haircut, especially when it's challenging. He taught me how to do tricks with the barber tools to get the haircut to come out the way the client wants.

And yes, I have pictures of me and the two inspirational barber teachers. They both definitely shaped my life in the barbershop world. I have much respect for these two barber teachers.

Watching the One Arm Barber work was like watching a magician. He'd position his client, position his tools, position his body in ways that compensated for having one arm. And the haircuts came out perfect. Every time. He showed me that limitations are just excuses. That if you want something bad enough, you'll find a way. Not an excuse. A way.

So let me tell you how I paid for the barber school. With all the side hustles of selling dinners on the weekend and doing cleanup jobs for my landlord and cleanup jobs for people in the same community. And my fiancée also helped me with the rest.

I managed to save up enough to get me in the barber school. And my fiancée put up the rest. Barber school cost about $5,000 at that time. I believe it's much more now.

Okay, so let me tell you the physical challenges while I was going to barber school and cutting hair. Yes, yes, it was very challenging.

Why I say this is because if you miss any days, you will have to make it up before graduating. So it takes six to nine months of barbering school. You must complete 900 hours of cutting hair. Cutting at least five hundred people, I believe, out of those nine hundred hours.

The school hours were from 9 AM to 2 PM Eastern Standard Time. It was a time in the morning hours when the weather was very bad. Cold. Windy. Raining. My lupus doesn't like bad weather.

So I had to come up with a remedy to get me through days like that and to perform haircuts on someone's hair.

So I did. I started eating a light breakfast and light lunch. My breakfast was a small cup of coffee, orange juice, and 2 slices of wheat bread. And my lunch was one slice wheat bread and a medium-size chicken cutlet with spinach.

I did this two hours ahead of time before going to the barber school. I did a lot of stretching and hand and wrist exercises. Because cutting hair takes a lot of hand and wrist work. So I did this routine the whole entire time going to the barber school.

Yes, sometimes it looked like it started not to work out for me on some days. Especially when it was snowing during winter. So I had to come up with something else so I don't miss no days of going to the school. Because I wanted to graduate on time.

So what I did was: While I was working on someone's haircut and my fingers would lock up because of the arthritis would kick in, I'd call one of the barber teachers to please take over for me because of my condition. And they understood.

What a release of stress off my mind and back.

So the barber teacher pulled me to the side and told me: "The number one rule in the school is, if you don't feel well or had a bad day at home, please do not cut anyone's hair. It's okay to sit on the side and still learn the education on how to cut hair."

I was so released of always trying to come up with a method to get through the day at the barber school. It was stressing me out to where I really didn't think I could make it all the way to the finish line. There were sleepless nights and worries in the morning.

But I ended up blessed with help from God and the teachers of the barber school. They saw me struggling. They saw me fighting through the pain. They saw me refusing to quit. And they said: "You don't have to prove anything to us. We already know you're strong. Now let us help you." And I let them. And that made all the difference.

I always felt the barbering and cooking was a good connection. Why I say this is because they both represent the word "good."

Food tastes good if you cook good. Haircuts come out good if you know how to cut good, especially when a person wants to look good. And that's why I chose that field of trades. I like to see people smile. I like to hear people tell me I did a good job on how I cut their hair, how I cooked the food they wanted and liked.

They both got a lot in common. Like they both represent some type of artwork. Artwork plays a part in a person's haircut, like when you're doing a specific style with different styles in the haircut. And when cooking food, you want the food to look like it tastes, with many styles of seasonings and colorful vegetables.

And it actually becomes everyone's style after a while. Just that everyone is different on how they do their own. This is the way I say they definitely have a connection between food and haircuts.

Both are about transformation. Both are about taking something raw and making it beautiful. Both are about making people feel good about themselves. Both are about service. About giving. About caring.

And so as you know, I did the exact same thing when it came down to preparing my food dish. I would master the combination of different herbs and spices. Sprinkling it on my meats and vegetables. Decorating my food like if I was doing artwork out of my food dish.

I would make sure my plate of food was full of many colorful fruits and vegetables. And the texture of the meat or poultry to blend right in perfectly.

I always try to make my food dish taste just how it looks. Pretty good and delicious.

How many times have you eaten at a restaurant or someone's house for dinner? Food looks so good. But the taste didn't match up. But you still force yourself to eat it. Or you will take it home and recook it, adding your own seasonings. That's disappointment. That's false advertising. That's not what I do. What you see is what you get. If it looks good, it tastes good. If it looks amazing, it tastes amazing. No surprises. No disappointments.

Once I saw how some people enjoyed my cooking and the food I would prepare for them, and they were admiring how I dress the plate with a style of colorful leafy salads and firm steamed veggies to juicy citrus fruits.

I used to see people take pictures of my dinners before eating it. And putting it up on social media and sending it to their friends.

So just to see that, it just gave me more encouragement, more aspiration to just keep at it and try to become the best at it. Because if people are taking pictures of your food before they eat it, that means you're doing something right. That means you're creating something worth documenting. Something worth sharing. Something beautiful.

So in my spare time, I would drive around my hometown cutting the homeless' hair for free and giving them a plate of food. Just to get that bright glow and smile of the day. To know that you made someone's day special. That was a true blessing to them and to me, knowing that I did that.

Because what's the point of having a skill if you don't use it to help people? What's the point of being blessed if you don't bless others? What's the point of surviving lupus if you don't use that survival to give hope to people who are barely surviving life?

Yes, this one particular homeless guy from the shelter did keep in touch, just for a little while. Only while I was still participating in the barber school.

Matter of fact, there were several people from the homeless shelter. It was about four gentlemen.

One was a motorcycle rider belonging to a motorcycle club in Brooklyn. Don't know the name, only what he told me.

One had just gotten out of a prison facility. He had done time like seventeen years in the prison.

One was a martial arts teacher in Harlem. He used to teach karate in a school until he lost everything. So now he started teaching people in the streets.

And there was another one who was a correction officer on Rikers Island.

They all kept coming to the barber school to see me on how I was making out and to get a haircut. And yes, I have pictures of all four, I believe.

These weren't just clients. These were connections. These were people who saw me struggling just like they were struggling. And we respected each other's struggle. We understood each other's pain. We didn't judge. We just helped.

The motorcycle rider would tell me stories about riding free on the open road before everything fell apart. The guy from prison would tell me about how hard it is to restart life when you lost seventeen years. The martial arts teacher would show me moves in the parking lot between haircuts. The correction officer would tell me about the other side of Rikers, about how easy it is to end up there if life goes wrong.

And I'd cut their hair. And feed them. And listen. Because sometimes that's all people need. Someone to see them. Someone to hear them. Someone to treat them like they matter. Because they do matter. Every single one of them matters.

So when I look back at that third-grade kid drawing cartoon characters, I see the beginning of everything. Art taught me to see. Not just to look, but to see. To see past the surface. To see what's underneath. To see the person behind the face. The story behind the smile. The pain behind the eyes.

And that's what barbering is. That's what cooking is. Both are about seeing people. About understanding what they need. About giving them something that makes them feel seen. Feel valued. Feel human.

A homeless man with crazy glue in his hair doesn't just need a haircut. He needs dignity. A professor who never had a haircut in sixty years doesn't just need a trim. He needs trust. A person eating your food doesn't just need nutrients. They need love. They need care. They need to know someone took time to make something beautiful just for them.

That's what my mom's artwork taught me. That's what Ms. Joseph taught me. That's what Mac at the barbershop taught me. That's what Mr. Dee and the One Arm

Barber taught me. That's what every homeless person I ever cut hair for taught me.

Art isn't about making pretty pictures. Art is about making people feel something. About changing something inside them. About giving them hope where there was none. About showing them beauty where they only saw ugliness. About proving to them they're worth the time. Worth the effort. Worth the care.

That's what I do. Whether I'm holding clippers or holding a spatula. Whether I'm cutting hair or cutting vegetables. Whether I'm blending a fade or blending spices. I'm creating art. And that art changes lives.

Because I've seen it happen. I've seen a man with crazy glue in his hair walk out with tears of gratitude. I've seen a professor with sixty years of uncut hair walk out looking 20 years younger. I've seen homeless men walk out standing taller, smiling brighter, believing again.

I've seen people take pictures of food before eating it because it's too beautiful to not document. I've seen people drive from Virginia for fish and grits. I've seen people's lives change because someone cared enough to make them something beautiful.

That's the craft I love most in my life. Not barbering. Not cooking. But transformation. Taking broken things and making them whole. Taking hurt people and giving them hope. Taking someone who gave up and showing them they still matter.

That's art. That's service. That's love. That's what God called me to do. And lupus can't stop that. Pain can't stop that. Arthritis in my fingers can't stop that. Nothing can stop that. Because it's not about me. It's about them. It's always been about them.

And as long as I have breath in my lungs and strength in my hands, I'll keep cutting hair. I'll keep cooking food. I'll keep creating art. I'll keep changing lives. One haircut at a time. One plate of food at a time. One person at a time.

Because that's what artists do. We don't just create beauty. We create hope. And this world needs all the hope it can get.

Chapter 12
From A Normal Life to A Life Living With Lupus

Yes, my lupus, my problem.

I am always thinking about what my life was like before I was diagnosed with systemic lupus. Was my body much stronger? Was my mindset much more successful? Or more focused?

Let's see. As I started thinking back in the day and years of my athletic life.

The answer is complicated. Because in some ways, yes, I was stronger. My body could do things then that it can't do now. But in other ways, no. Because lupus forced me to become strong in ways I never had to be before. Mental strength. Spiritual strength. The strength to keep going when your body is screaming at you to stop.

I remember I used to get up in the morning to go jogging like it was mandatory before starting my day. I would go to work after a two-hour run. And work an eight-hour shift. In between I'd take short ten-minute breaks and workout by doing pushups and pullups. And I would do this six times before my eight-hour shift was over with.

And when I got off, I would go to the boxing gym and workout some more for two hours. Jumping rope. And doing sit-ups. And spar people in the ring for six or seven rounds.

And when I finally got home and showered up and rested a bit, I'd do another hour workout by punching the heavy bag and doing pushups and dips. And I was doing this same routine from the age of twelve to age twenty-four.

Let me break down exactly what a typical day looked like:

6 AM: Wake up. Get dressed. Head to Paterson, New Jersey, East Side Park. That's a well-known park in the city of Paterson. All Paterson special events are given there. Including people who give family gatherings. Also state carnival fairs for kids in the community. The park holds about thirty to forty blocks.

So I used to go jogging up at that park for three hours nonstop. Three hours. Not walking. Not jogging and walking. Running. For three hours straight. That's the kind of conditioning I had. That's the kind of machine my body was.

9 AM: After jogging, I'd workout on the park monkey bars. Which is the bars all the kids can play on, swinging upside down and walking across with their body hanging down with their hands. Those bars we called monkey bars.

So I used to then go there after jogging for three hours. And I'd do thirty sets of twenty-five pullups, front and back ways. I'd do twenty sets of twenty leg lifts.

Think about that math. Thirty sets of twenty-five pullups. That's seven hundred and fifty pullups. Twenty sets of twenty leg lifts. That's four hundred leg lifts. After running for three hours. That's not normal. That's obsession. That's dedication. That's a machine.

10:30 AM: After the monkey bars, it used to be others who were working out up at the park also. So it used to be a circle stage in the middle of the park where me and the guys up at the park used to do some boxing sparring with the boxing gloves.

I used to carry my boxing equipment in the trunk of my car. Because after a workout, I needed to spar. Some guys I knew personally. And some guys I just met. And so we used to work out with the gloves on for about two hours.

But let me make it clear: I would never stop the whole two hours. Only when it was time for another one of the guys to put on the boxing gloves, the other guy took off. See, what's going on is I'd spar eight to ten different guys, one at a time. Because that was my workout.

But some guys were skillful. And some guys wanted to see if I really knew how to box. And some guys just wanted to learn.

12:30 PM: After I was finished up there, when it wasn't no one left to workout with the boxing gloves, I would then go to work. And work an eight-hour shift.

But I'd also workout in between the hours until getting off of work. Me and some of the other employees at the job would have pushup contests and pullup contests.

And I had a close friend whose name was Graham. We were like brothers. We were very close. Did everything the same.

We used to both box at the same gym. We both have the same birthday. We both were mommy's boys. We both hung out after work and weekends.

So anyway, we both had a thing where we would always have to test each other's boxing skills so often. So every day at work, we would spar with the boxing gloves and without the boxing gloves. And it used to be rough.

But we never got serious to where we became enemies or got into real fights with each other. Because we had a personal bond to where whoever wins in a boxing match that day, we cannot get upset. Some days it will be my day to win or your day to win.

And we did not let anyone come between us to make us turn against each other. That was our code. That was our brotherhood. Nobody could break that.

8:30 PM: So this part of a routine of workouts would be an everyday thing for me. I'd workout at the park and at work with friends. And I'd workout more after work in my home on the basketball courts.

I'd jog around the basketball courts ten times while dribbling the basketball. And then I'd shoot some hoops with some guys who were out there on the courts or by myself. And I'd do that for two hours.

10:30 PM: And after I finished with that, I'd go in the back of the basketball courts and get on the pullup bars and do twenty sets of twenty pullups and dips.

And then go in the house and punch my heavy punching bag I had in my room hanging from my closet. My homemade boxing gym in my house.

So I'd punch the bag for forty minutes. And then I'd do some bench press with two-hundred-pound weights. And I'd do that for forty minutes, ten times of lifting.

And once I'm finished, I'd take my shower and go to bed. And get ready to do the same routine the next day.

I was always looking forward to doing the same workouts every day. I was a workout fanatic. Anywhere I was and I had spare time, I would workout. Doing pullups and dips and pushups.

And driving around to some of the blocks in the neighborhood with the boxing gloves in my car just to workout with some of the guys.

But it came to a point of time where I had to pay money to older guys who were kind of much more experienced than I was to workout with me with the boxing gloves.

And these guys were serious ex-professional street fighters. Without the gloves and with the gloves. They knew how to fight on a professional level. Like if they were in a boxing ring or if they were in a street fight. To be clear on that.

So yes, I was on a mission of learning all different types and styles of the boxing game and mixing it up into my own styles. See, that's what all of us do that love that type of sport.

So basically, I worked out every day, all day, if I could, before being diagnosed with lupus.

I mean, some people used to get mad at me when they saw me coming around. Because they knew I was going to ask them to workout with me. Especially with the boxing gloves.

I was determined to be good and get good at it. I was definitely dreaming of becoming professional one day. But not for a career. I kind of wanted to see if I could really do it. Make it in the boxing sport.

I ended up making it to the summer tournaments, the Golden Gloves. That would go on every year.

First was the amateur fight night at a high school gym in Newark, New Jersey. And then a couple of weeks later, there was the Golden Gloves in Paterson, New Jersey, St. Mary's Church community hall.

So let me be specific and clear: You would have to fight in the amateur fight night two to three times before entering the Golden Gloves. And you have to win, I believe, also both fights. Three-minute rounds with eight-ounce gloves.

It's like fighting with your bare knuckles. Because we spar with 16-ounce gloves when working out at the boxing gym. So eight-ounce gloves feel like nothing. Every punch lands hard. Every hit you feel.

So anyway, I won my first two amateur fights. And went on to Golden Gloves.

But let me tell you exactly what happened.

My first fight, I won by TKO in the first round. Technical knockout. I dominated. I was fast. I was powerful. I was in the zone. The other guy couldn't keep up. The ref stopped it. Victory.

Number two fight, I won in round two out of three rounds we were supposed to do.

But they took the win of the fight from me. Because I was on medications. Muscle relaxers.

See, I was doing too much training for the tournaments. To where I over-trained. And I pulled some muscles between my groin area from too much jogging. And had to go to the hospital and get checked out.

And that was the problem. I pulled some muscles. They prescribed me some muscle relaxers and told me to rest for a couple of weeks.

So me being a stubborn person, I didn't. Because I wanted to be in that tournament so desperately.

So no, I didn't listen to the doctors. I entered the tournament while taking a muscle relaxer. And thinking everything would be okay.

But once the muscle relaxer kicked in, they recognized that something was wrong. But after I won the boxing match.

And the judges at the tournaments had me checked out by their doctors to see for any hyped-up drugs. And when they did, they discovered I was on muscle relaxers.

And they said to me and the judges: "Just because he was on any form of a drug or meds at the time of the tournament, we will have to strip him of the win of the fight."

And gave it to the other guy who I won the fight against.

I was so brokenhearted that I didn't want to even box no more at all. I trained so hard. I won fair and square. And they took it from me because I was trying to push through an injury. Because I wanted it so bad.

So once I entered the Golden Gloves, I had to fight a guy who was about to turn professional in six months.

People at the tournaments said, "That's not right. That's not an even match-up."

But my boxing coaches from my gym said, "It's okay. He's good. We believe he's ready."

So I did fight the soon-to-be professional boxer in the first round.

But when the second round started, I stopped. I decided not to go on.

Let me tell you why.

One of my coaches from the gym said something to me that turned me off from participating anymore in the tournament. Before going back into the middle of the ring, he whispered into my ear:

"If you don't win this fight, do not come back to my boxing gym."

I was hurt. Wondering: Why would you say that to me? Is this how you feel about me? I am just a piece of fighting garbage? A machine you must be making money bets on?

So when the bell rang, I turned around and gave up the fight. Letting the other guy take the win.

So for the record, I never took a loss in the boxing tournaments. I gave the loss because of how I was treated.

That coach didn't see me as a person. He saw me as an investment. A way to make money. And the minute I wasn't going to win, I was worthless to him. That hurt worse than any punch I ever took.

So for the record, yes, my boxing record was: one TKO, one draw, one loss. Because I gave up the win for a loss.

But to me, I was three fights, no losses. To me.

Because I didn't lose those fights. I won one. They took one from me. And I walked away from one. None of those are real losses. Those are circumstances. Those are other people's decisions. Not my ability failing.

So as times moved on, I stopped going to that particular gym in my neighborhood.

Meanwhile, I'm searching for other gyms to join. One of my brothers, who goes by the name Sneak a Peak, well, because I wasn't going to a gym at the time, he started to teach me how he got good with boxing.

He himself showed me all he knows. With street boxing to ring boxing.

A popular street boxing style everyone will always know my brother for was called trick boxing. It was a boxing style where you can outthink your opponents in any style of fighting.

And when he couldn't teach me no more new tricks in the boxing sport, he then took me around my hometown of Paterson, New Jersey, to some of his friends. Some the same age. Some just a little older.

That had taught him how to box in the ring and in the streets. And these guys were nowhere in shape. But still knew how to fight really good.

They don't workout anymore and not 100 percent healthy-wise. But natural-gifted fighters in the boxing game.

When he took me to get trained by these different friends of his, he told them to teach me like they taught him. And that meant: Do not take it easy on me. I must learn what it takes to be a smart fighter. A strong fighter. And a tough fighter. Because in this boxing game, it's full of surprises. And you never know what you're going to get in the ring.

These men beat me up. Not to hurt me. But to teach me. They'd hit me hard and say, "See? That's what happens when you drop your guard." They'd fake left and go right and say, "See? That's what happens when you don't watch the hips." They taught me through pain. Through repetition. Through making me feel what would happen if I made mistakes in a real fight.

And I started to slow down a bit. And I started doing less reps and sets. And skipping a lot of days where I felt like I was getting bored with working out. Or just becoming lazy.

I know once I started to pay bills, my lifestyle of living took a toll on me. Like my rent. My public service. Phone bills. Gas and maintenance on the car.

So as I got more and more into trying to maintain my bills and keeping a job, my exercising habits changed to where I only worked out either in the morning for two to three hours or at night before going to bed, two to three hours.

My meals before lupus were the average. I'd eat two to three bowls of cereal or oatmeal for breakfast. For lunch, I'd have a full ten-inch sub sandwich. For dinner, I'd have some fried chicken and rice and vegetables. And a couple of snacks like potato chips or a bowl of grapes or a Snickers bar or some banana pudding.

I was eating to fuel a machine. That's what my body was. A machine that needed constant fuel. I wasn't thinking about nutrition. I was thinking about calories. About energy. About keeping the engine running.

How much did I weigh at the time of being into sports? I weighed about a hundred and seventy-eight pounds. That also was my boxing class weight.

Now I weigh about two hundred and ten pounds. Thirty-two pounds heavier. But not from muscle. From medication. From inactivity. From my body changing in ways I couldn't control.

And after time went on, my appetite started to change also. Didn't feel like eating healthy foods or vegetables. Just a lot of cereal. And drinking a lot of sugary juices.

So as I went for my regular doctor's visits, I explained to my doctor how I'd been feeling lately. And about how certain things changed with my eating habits and exercises. How I don't have an appetite for food or energy to workout. And when I do eat, I eat very little. And workout very little. And my muscles get really sore quickly. And I'm always tired and out of breath.

So my doctors ran a couple of lab tests. And after a few years, my doctors discovered I have systemic lupus.

So as they explained to me how it works, and there's no cure for lupus, just to treat it and keep it stable, stay on track with doctor's appointments and keep up with all medications. And I did just that.

And the physical side of my body changes when becoming sick was a strange feeling type. Like I just didn't have the urge of working out long or working out every day. My body started to feel weak and out of tune. My muscles were always hurting. I started getting tired too fast. A lot of activities just didn't feel the same anymore. I just started having no more interest in doing nothing but going to work.

It's hard to explain to someone who's never been athletic. Imagine you're a car. And you've always been a race car. Fast. Powerful. Responsive. And then one day, you wake up and you're a regular car. Not broken. Just regular. The engine still runs. But it's not the same engine. It doesn't respond the same. It doesn't have the same power. That's what it felt like. Like someone swapped out my engine while I was sleeping.

The time I found out I couldn't do the same physical activities anymore is when I couldn't run a full lap around the park. When I couldn't do many pushups and pullups and dips.

I can tell you the time my body failed me is when I was working out at the gym and me and this guy were boxing. And I couldn't be as skillful as I knew I was. Like I just forgot how to box anymore.

And my body was hurting quickly as the guy punched my body. I gave up quickly. That's when I knew my body was failing me.

I remember that moment so clearly. This guy wasn't even good. I should have been able to handle him easy. But my hands were slow. My feet were slow. My reflexes were gone. And every punch he landed hurt more than it should have. Not because he was hitting harder. But because my body couldn't take it anymore. Couldn't absorb it. Couldn't bounce back.

And I stopped. And I took off the gloves. And I walked out of that gym. And I never went back.

Because I knew. I knew it was over. I knew the athlete I was, was gone. And I didn't know what I was going to be instead.

But as time went on, I started to discover side effects the doctors didn't know about. So I tried doing my own studies on lupus. And tried coming up with a solution to maintain it to make me feel as normal as possible. Not take all these meds and me feel like a whole different person.

I mean, the meds made me feel like sleeping all day. Hungry all the time. Some meds always gave me headaches. Or made me itch like crazy.

So I tried concentrating on: What can I do to try to get my normal life back?

I started studying fruits and vegetables that meet some of the medications as a substitute. I also studied the right herbs and spices for poultry and light meats. Like chicken or turkey. Not too much beef or pork. I had to cut that out of my life entirely, almost.

It was so much to deal with trying to maintain this lupus on natural treatment substances.

And once I got to realize that, I knew I had to get stronger physically and mentally. Most everything I do had to become a project and a mission in my life.

Because the doctors could only do so much. The medications helped. But they also hurt. So I had to find my own way. I had to become my own scientist. My own nutritionist. My own coach. I had to figure out what worked for my body. What didn't. What helped. What made it worse.

I'll tell you the thing I miss most about my normal life is working a nine to five. Claiming income tax at the end of the year.

I miss being able to just get up in the morning and just get dressed and eat a big breakfast and start my day without the meds.

I miss playing sports. Especially boxing. Basketball.

I miss the feeling of pushing my body to its limits and knowing it will respond. I miss the confidence of knowing I can do anything physically. I miss the competition. The adrenaline. The feeling of winning.

I miss looking in the mirror and seeing an athlete. Seeing someone strong. Seeing someone capable.

Now when I look in the mirror, I see someone surviving. And that's important. Survival is important. But it's not the same as thriving. It's not the same as being in your prime. It's not the same as feeling invincible.

My mental toughness from boxing helped me fight lupus. On the fact that I just wanted my life to still go on. I still wanted to live life. I still wanted to be a part of the world. I couldn't sit around feeling sorry for myself. It just didn't feel right.

I built up my toughness mentally by watching others who were in a worse suffering condition than I was in. As I watch the advertisement commercials of the St. Jude kids with special needs on TV.

By the way, I've been donating to that organization, to their hospital, for many years before lupus.

Anyway, I spent time talking to homeless, handicapped, and disabled people in the streets who have no one to help them at all. Family-wise or friend-wise.

I think about the fallen Army soldiers and disabled veterans who've been tossed to the streets.

I think about the babies who were born with many health issues.

I think about all kids who have to spend the rest of their lives in a hospital.

This is how, then and now, to this day, I keep my mental strong and tough.

Boxing taught me: You're going to get hit. That's guaranteed. The question is: What do you do after you get hit? Do you quit? Do you cry? Do you give up? Or do you get back up? Do you adjust? Do you find a way to win anyway?

Lupus hit me hard. Knocked me down. Took away everything I thought I was. But boxing taught me how to get back up. How to adjust my strategy. How to find a way to win even when the odds are against me.

Every round in boxing is three minutes. And you just have to survive those three minutes. Then you get a break. Then you go again. That's how I treat lupus. Day by day. Round by round. Just survive today. Just get through this flare. Just make it to the next doctor's appointment. And then rest. And then go again.

So as I said before: Normal life versus life with lupus. Which one you think made me stronger as a person?

Even though I was doing a lot of things that would still help me in my life, like work and workout, pay my bills, eat okay foods. But when discovering I have lupus, it made me want to get smarter and take my life a lot more seriously on the healthy side. By studying every food diet to keep me strong. And every workout to keep me fit.

So I don't quit on trying to find the right lifestyle to fit my new life now that I will have to share it with systemic lupus.

Here's what I learned:

Normal life made me physically strong. But life with lupus made me mentally strong. Spiritually strong. Emotionally strong.

Normal life taught me how to win. But life with lupus taught me how to survive. How to keep going when winning isn't possible. How to find purpose when your body fails you. How to redefine success. How to measure victory in getting out of bed. In taking your meds. In making it through the day.

Normal life gave me confidence. But life with lupus gave me humility. It taught me I'm not invincible. It taught me I'm not in control. It taught me to appreciate every good day. Every moment without pain. Every small victory.

Normal life taught me to push through pain. But life with lupus taught me to listen to pain. To respect it. To understand it's my body's way of saying slow down. Rest. Take care of yourself.

Normal life taught me to be tough. But life with lupus taught me to be gentle. With myself. With my limitations. With my new reality.

So which made me stronger? Both. In different ways. I needed both. I needed the athlete I was to survive becoming the person I am. I needed the discipline. The work ethic. The mental toughness. The refusal to quit. All of that came from my athletic life. And all of that saved me when lupus tried to destroy me.

If I could go back and tell myself before having lupus, it would be this:

Always be thankful for life. Because you never know of the unexpected challenges in life. You never know what the future holds. Especially for someone who was in the best of shape.

So always be mindful. Try in so many ways to monitor your whole entire life. Life itself can always be full of mysteries.

I would tell myself: Take pictures of yourself at your peak. Write down how it feels to be strong. Remember every moment. Because one day, you'll want to remember what that felt like.

I would tell myself: Be kind to your body. Yes, push it. Yes, train hard. But also listen to it. Rest when it needs rest. Don't over-train. Don't ignore injuries. Don't think you're invincible.

I would tell myself: Your body is not your identity. You are more than an athlete. You are more than your physical abilities. So when those abilities are taken away, you'll still be you. You'll still have value. You'll still have purpose.

I would tell myself: Don't take any day for granted. Not the hard training days. Not the competition days. Not even the rest days. Because one day, you'll wish you could have just one more training day. Just one more fight. Just one more moment of feeling strong.

I would tell myself: Boxing will teach you everything you need to know to survive lupus. The discipline. The mental toughness. The ability to get hit and keep going. The understanding that some fights you lose. But you never quit. You never give up. You always show up for the next round.

But most of all, I would tell myself: You're going to be okay. It won't feel like it. It'll feel like your life is over. It'll feel like you've lost everything. But you haven't. You've just lost one version of yourself. And you'll build a new version. A different version. Not weaker. Just different.

And that version will be strong too. Just in ways you can't imagine yet. Ways that don't require 750 pullups or three-hour runs or sparring sessions. Ways that require waking up when your body is screaming. Taking meds that make you sick. Going to appointments. Cooking healing food. Stretching aching joints. Finding joy in small victories.

That's strength too. Maybe even greater strength. Because anybody can be strong when their body cooperates. But being strong when your body betrays you? That takes something special. That takes heart. That takes faith. That takes the kind of toughness you can't build in a gym.

And you have that toughness. You've always had it. You just didn't know it yet. Because you didn't need it yet. But when you do need it, it'll be there. And you'll survive. And you'll find a way to keep fighting. Because that's what fighters do. They fight. No matter what. No matter the odds. No matter the opponent.

And lupus is just another opponent. A tough one. Maybe the toughest you'll ever face. But you'll face it. And you'll find a way to live with it. And you'll keep your head to the sky. And you'll keep moving forward. One day at a time. One round at a time. Until the final bell.

That's what I would tell my pre-lupus self. And I hope he'd listen. But knowing him, probably not. He was too stubborn. Too confident. Too sure of his invincibility. Just like I needed him to be. Just like he needed to be to survive what was coming.

Because maybe you have to believe you're invincible before you can learn that you're not. Maybe you have to be broken before you can be remade into something stronger. Maybe you have to lose everything before you can appreciate what you still have.

Maybe that's the real lesson. Not normal life versus life with lupus. But normal life preparing you for life with lupus. Normal life giving you the tools you'd need to survive life with lupus. Normal life building the foundation that life with lupus would test.

And I'm still here. Still fighting. Still standing. Thirty-two pounds heavier. A lot slower. A lot weaker physically. But still here. Still moving. Still finding ways to work out. Still finding ways to help people. Still finding ways to matter.

That's my victory. Not a TKO in the first round. Not a championship belt. Not a perfect record. Just survival. Just persistence. Just refusing to quit when everything in me wanted to.

That's what athletes do. We don't quit. We adjust. We adapt. We overcome. We find a way.

And I found a way. It's not the way I planned. It's not the way I wanted. But it's my way. And it's enough.

That's my lupus. That's my problem. That's my fight. And I'm still in the ring. Still throwing punches. Still believing I can win. Maybe not by knockout. Maybe just by decision. Maybe just by surviving all the rounds. But winning nonetheless.

Because I'm still here. And as long as I'm still here, the fight's not over. And as long as the fight's not over, I've still got a chance. And as long as I've got a chance, I'm going to keep fighting.

That's what my normal life taught me. That's what my life with lupus reinforced. That's what I carry with me every single day.

Keep fighting. Keep moving. Keep believing. Keep your head to the sky.

Because the bell hasn't rung yet. And until it does, I'm still in this fight.

Chapter 13
A Couple of Dreams I Had Before I Got Lupus

When you're young, you dream big.

Let me start from the time in my youth years of playing sports.

I loved basketball, though I was not too good at it. I loved football, though I was okay in it. I liked playing baseball, but not as a professional.

But when I was introduced to boxing, I saw, and others that saw me saw, that I had a little talent and skills in it. And I fell in love with it very quickly.

Especially as I started to know about all the famous professional fighters. Like Muhammad Ali. Joe Frazier. George Foreman. And my favorite, the one and only Evander Holyfield.

These weren't just boxers to me. They were heroes. They were proof that you could come from nothing and become somebody that is really big in the boxing game. They showed me that hard work and dedication could take you anywhere. That if you were willing to bleed and sweat and sacrifice, you could make it to the top.

Holyfield especially. The way he fought. The way he never gave up. The way he came back from losses stronger than before. That's who I wanted to be. That's who I thought I could be.

I started boxing at one of the youth gyms in my hometown of Paterson, New Jersey. And I became popular with it. Because some of the people who were at the same gym would spread the word around my hometown.

And people started to come to the gym to watch me spar in the boxing ring. All the way until I was entering the Golden Gloves and Diamond Gloves tournaments.

That feeling when people come just to watch you train? That's something special. That's validation. That's proof you're not wasting your time. That what you're doing matters. That you're good at something. Really good.

I remember looking up from the ring and seeing people lined up at the ropes. Watching. Nodding. Talking to each other. Pointing. "That's him. That's Pretty Boy. Watch this." And I'd throw my signature one-two punch. And they'd react. And I'd feel ten feet tall.

The boxing tournaments were so fun. Especially when your hometown is shouting your name and rooting for you.

I just knew I was going to take it. I just knew I was going to become a professional.

That wasn't hope. That wasn't a wish. That was certainty. That was knowing. I could feel it in my bones. I could see it in my future. Professional boxer. Fighting on TV. Making money. Making my family proud. Making Paterson proud. That was my destiny. That's what I was born to do.

My best boxing match was my first boxing match in the boxing tournament. The boxing match only went one round.

I punched the guy so hard, so many times at once, his headgear popped off of him.

As the referee stopped the fight to fix my opponent's headgear and they restarted the fight, I then punched my opponent to the stomach area. And he dropped to his knees. And couldn't get back up.

So they ended the fight with a TKO. Stands for technical knockout.

Let me walk you through it because that moment is burned into my memory. That moment is everything I was. Everything I could have been.

The bell rings. We touch gloves. Circle each other. He throws a jab. I slip it. He throws another. I slip that too. I'm faster than him. I can see it in his eyes. He knows it too.

Then I see my opening. He drops his right hand just a little. Just for a second. But that's all I need.

I throw my signature one-two. Left jab to set it up. Right hand to finish it. Clean. Hard. Fast. The jab snaps his head back. The right hand lands flush on his temple. His legs wobble. His eyes glaze.

The crowd erupts. "Pretty Boy! Pretty Boy! Pretty Boy!"

I don't stop. I can't stop. This is what I trained for. This is what all those hours in the gym were for. All those early mornings. All those sparring sessions. All that pain. For this moment.

I throw another combination. Jab, jab, right hand. All three land. His headgear flies off. Just pops right off his head and lands on the canvas.

The ref steps in. Stops the fight. Picks up the headgear. Puts it back on my opponent's head. Checks him. "You okay? You want to continue?" My opponent nods. But I can see it. He doesn't want to continue. He's done. He just doesn't know it yet.

The ref signals to restart. And I know what I have to do. End it. Don't let him suffer. Don't drag this out. Respect him by finishing him quickly.

We restart. He's cautious now. Protecting his head. Hands high. Chin tucked. So I go to the body.

I throw a left hook to his ribs. He grunts. I throw a right uppercut to his solar plexus. All the air leaves his body. His hands drop. His knees buckle. He drops.

The ref counts. One. Two. Three. My opponent tries to get up. Four. Five. He's on one knee. Six. Seven. He's trying. But his body won't cooperate. Eight. Nine. Ten.

TKO. Technical knockout. I win.

The crowd goes crazy. My corner rushes the ring. My coach hugs me. "That's my boy! That's my fighter!" I raise my hands. The ref raises my hand. I look out at the crowd and see all my homeboys from my block, cheering for me and it felt good.

That moment. That feeling. That's what I chased for years. That's what I thought my life would be. Professional boxer. Champion. Holyfield 2.0.

My boxing nickname was Pretty Boy. Killer with the right-hand punch.

My one and two punch was my boxing style. Two punches was my signature boxing style I was known for. It was almost always over with those two punches.

People would come to see if they could handle my one-two. And most couldn't. That right hand came so fast. And it came so hard. And once it landed, the fight was usually over. Or the beginning of the end.

They called me Pretty Boy because I didn't have a lot of scars. Like a lot of fighters you usually see, and I always was trying to look handsome for the ladies. Because I didn't get hit much. I was too fast. Too slick. Too good defensively. I'd slip punches. Dodge punches. Make guys miss. Then counter with my one-two. And good-night.

That was my style. Hit and don't get hit. Make you miss. Make you pay. One-two. It's over.

The professional boxers I got to meet were a couple from my hometown. It was about six professionals I was kind of close to, by the names S Sharp, T Money, B Boy, Master King, JJ, Mack T, Shock G.

And I also still sometimes see these guys in the streets. Who still are active in the gym at the age of 65 and 68.

And that is another one of my inspirations in life. To stay fighting hard mentally and physically and spiritually.

These weren't celebrities to me. These were neighbors. These were guys from my block. My town. My gym. Guys who made it. Who fought on TV. Who made money. Who proved it was possible.

I'd see them at the gym. Training. Even after they retired. Even at sixty and sixty-five. Still in shape. Still throwing punches. Still sharp. Still relevant. Still fighters.

And they'd give me advice. "Keep your hands up." "Work the body." "Don't get lazy." "Stay hungry." "The minute you think you've made it, that's when you lose it." Real advice from real fighters who lived it.

That's what I wanted. That longevity. That respect. That legacy. To be 65 and still relevant. Still training. Still inspiring the next generation. Still being Pretty Boy. Just older. Wiser. But still a fighter.

What ended my boxing dreams was knowing lupus would not allow me to participate in that type of physical activity anymore.

After doing my research and dealing with lupus and varicose veins causing me to always be in the hospital or on bed rest, I just knew it was time to let go of that dream.

That's the hardest sentence I've ever had to write. "It was time to let go of that dream."

Because that dream wasn't just a dream. It was my identity. It was who I was. It was my future. My purpose. My reason for waking up at 5 AM. My reason for pushing through pain. My reason for everything.

And lupus took it. Just like that. Not all at once. But slowly. Gradually. My stamina went first. Couldn't spar as many rounds. Then my power went. Punches didn't land as hard. Then my speed went. Couldn't slip punches like before. Then my recovery went. Body hurt for days after training instead of hours.

And then came the varicose veins. Legs swelling so bad I couldn't train. Couldn't run. Could barely walk. In and out of the hospital. Bed rest. Medications. More bed rest. More medications.

And I had to face the truth: I couldn't be a professional boxer. My body wouldn't let me. Lupus wouldn't let me. And no amount of heart or determination or wanting it bad enough could change that.

So I let it go. Not because I wanted to. But because I had to. Because holding onto a dream that's impossible only makes you suffer. Only makes you bitter. Only makes you angry at the world.

So I let it go. And I cried. And I mourned. And I grieved the loss of Pretty Boy the boxer. And then I started figuring out who Johnny with lupus could be instead.

I remember when I started one of my first jobs at a fast food restaurant. And how I started to learn to cook all types of food and became good at it. I saw I had a gift within it. And it made me feel good. And it was lots of fun doing it.

I started to add this to my "I have a dream" plan of owning my own restaurant one day. Especially once I knew how much money you can make.

The first day I worked at a fast food restaurant, it was Wendy's.

I learned how to flip the perfect hamburger. And I learned how to make my favorite food from scratch: beef chili and cheese.

They showed me how to make it out of hamburger meat with peppers and onions and spices. And it always came out good. And I still do it that way.

That first day, I was nervous. I'd never worked in a kitchen before. Never cooked professionally. I could cook at home. But this was different. This was fast. This was under pressure. This was for customers who were paying money and expecting quality.

My trainer that day was this older lady named Miss Rosa. She'd been working at Wendy's for fifteen years. Knew everything. Seen everything. Could work every station with her eyes closed.

She showed me the grill. "This is where you'll spend most of your time. Burgers go on here. You don't move them. You don't press them. You don't touch them until it's time to flip. You flip once. Only once. Too many flips, you lose the juice. You lose the flavor."

I watched her. She made it look easy. Burgers on the grill. Sizzling. Smoking. The smell filling the kitchen. Timer goes off. Flip. All of them. One smooth motion. Like a dance. Timer goes off again. Off the grill. Onto the buns. To the assembly line.

"Your turn," she said.

My hands were shaking. I put the burgers on the grill. Waited. Timer went off. I flipped. But I wasn't smooth like her. I fumbled. Hesitated. But I got them flipped.

"Not bad," she said. "You'll get faster. You'll get smoother. Just takes practice. Just like anything else."

And she was right. By the end of that first shift, I was faster. Smoother. More confident. And I realized: I liked this. I liked cooking. I liked the heat. The pressure. The rhythm. The satisfaction of making something people enjoyed.

And then Miss Rosa showed me the chili. How to brown the meat. How to drain the fat. How to add the peppers, the onions, the spices. How to let it simmer. How to taste it. How to adjust.

"Cooking is about more than following a recipe," she said. "It's about tasting. Adjusting. Making it yours. This is Wendy's chili. But when you make it, it becomes your chili. Because you're the one who tasted it. Adjusted it. Made it right."

That lesson stuck with me. That's why when I cook now, I taste. I adjust. I make it mine. Because Miss Rosa taught me: cooking is personal. Cooking is art. Even at Wendy's. Even with fast food. There's still art in it. There's still you in it.

My signature dish from those restaurant days was BBQ chicken and candied yams and macaroni and cheese. And that was my favorite for many years.

That meal right there? That's soul food. That's comfort. That's home. That's love on a plate.

The BBQ chicken I learned from working at different places after Wendy's. How to season it. How to grill it. How to baste it with sauce so it gets that caramelized crust but stays juicy inside.

The candied yams I learned from my mom. How to peel them. Slice them. Layer them in the pan with butter and brown sugar and cinnamon and a little nutmeg. How to bake them until they're soft and sweet and the syrup is thick and bubbly.

The mac and cheese I learned by trial and error. Trying different cheeses. Different ratios. Different techniques. Until I found the perfect combination: sharp cheddar for flavor. Mild cheddar for creaminess. A little cream cheese for smoothness. Baked until the top is golden and crispy but the inside is creamy and cheesy.

Put those three together on a plate, and people's eyes light up. They see it and they know: this is going to be good. This is real food. This is made with care. This is made with love.

That's the meal I became known for. That's the meal people would request. "Johnny, when you making that chicken and yams and mac again?" That's the meal that made me think: I could do this professionally. I could open a restaurant. This could be my new dream.

But as time went on and seeing how my life started to change and transform to where I couldn't perform certain physical activities in the sports world, I had to change up a lot of my dreams to where it wouldn't involve too much physical activity.

So I thought about being an interior designer. Party promoter. Then at last, a professional barber.

So I decided to go to school and get my master's degree in master barber.

And hopefully I can break into the movies and commercials, music and videos. And cut and groom the actors in those types of lifeline industry circuits. In a way, even until today, I'm still trying for that particular dream.

Here's what happened:

When I realized boxing was over, I went through a list. What can I do that doesn't require peak physical condition? What can I do that uses my talents but works around my limitations?

Interior designer: I've always been good with colors. With arranging things. With making spaces look good. Maybe I could do that professionally. Design homes. Design offices. Design restaurants.

But that requires a lot of standing. A lot of measuring. A lot of lifting. And with my legs, with the varicose veins, with the lupus flares, I knew that would be hard to sustain.

Party promoter: I'm good with people. I know how to hype things up. How to get people excited. How to spread the word. Maybe I could promote parties. Promote events. Promote clubs.

But that requires a lot of late nights. A lot of standing. A lot of physical energy. And with lupus, my energy is unpredictable. Some days I have it. Some days I don't. Can't build a business on unpredictability.

Professional barber: I'm already cutting hair. Already good at it. Already have clients. Already have the artistic eye from drawing as a kid. Already have the people skills from boxing and promoting myself. This could work. This could actually work.

So I went to barber school. Got my master barber license. Started building a clientele. Started perfecting my craft. Started seeing this as more than a job. Started seeing this as my new dream.

Cut hair for celebrities. For actors. For musicians. For athletes. Be the barber people request by name. Be the barber who shows up on set. Who travels with the talent. Who gets credited in the thank you's. That could be my new version of success. My new version of making it.

Yes, I am still keeping my dreams of being in movies, commercials, and modeling.

I recently just took a couple of modeling photoshoots. I am signed up with a modeling photo company called Maps Models.

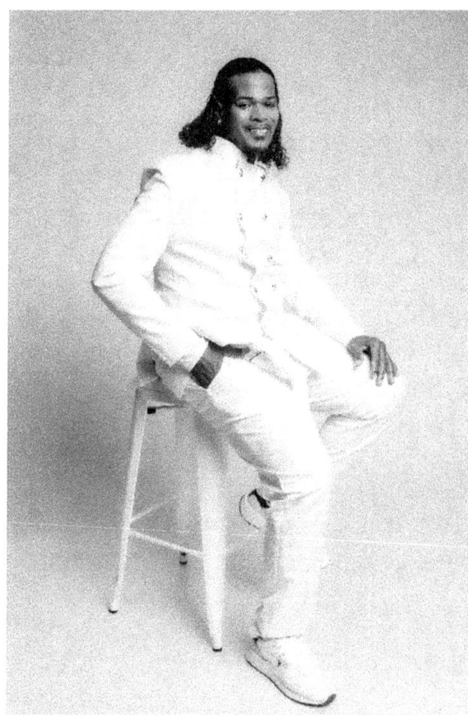

I am hopefully going to get the attention of some movie producers and hopefully get to appear on Netflix or Amazon movies.

So yes, I am still pursuing my movies and TV commercials dreams.

Yes, I did. I took steps by trying to build up my portfolio with Maps Models in NYC of Manhattan.

I went online and put my information into a lot of audition websites. And I'm still looking to get into other connections related.

People ask me: "Aren't you too old to start modeling and acting?" And I say: "Too old according to who? I'm still here. I still look good. I still have something to offer. And until they tell me no, I'm going to keep trying."

Because here's what lupus taught me: dreams don't die unless you kill them. They transform. They adapt. They change shape. But they don't die.

I can't be a professional boxer. But I can be a barber who cuts professional boxers' hair.

I can't own a restaurant yet. But I can cook professionally and sell my food and build toward that.

I can't be Muhammad Ali. But I can be in a commercial. I can be in a movie. I can be on Netflix. Different dream. Same feeling. Same success. Just a different path.

So I'm building my portfolio. Taking photoshoots. Submitting to casting calls. Networking. Connecting. Putting myself out there. Because the only way you definitely don't make it is by not trying.

And I'm not ready to stop trying. Lupus slowed me down. But it didn't stop me. And as long as I'm not stopped, I'm still in the game. Still in the fight. Still chasing dreams.

If I could design my perfect day of work right now, it would be like this:

I'd be at work. And everything with everyone I'm working with would run smoothly without any situations. And I'd just know I'm getting a raise in my salary.

But let me expand on that. Because that's the practical answer. Here's the dream answer:

My perfect day starts at 8 AM. Not 5 AM like when I was boxing. But 8 AM. A reasonable hour for a body with lupus.

I wake up without pain. Without stiffness. Without that heavy feeling that makes getting out of bed feel like climbing a mountain. I wake up feeling good. Feeling rested. Feeling ready.

I take my meds with a good breakfast. Not rushed. Not stressed. Just calm. Peaceful. Starting the day right.

By 9 AM, I'm in my own barbershop. Not working for someone else. My own shop. My name on the door. My vision. My space. Clean. Professional. Welcoming. Music playing. Earth, Wind & Fire. "Keep Your Head to the Sky."

My first client arrives at 9:30. He's an actor. Or a musician. Or an athlete. Someone whose work I respect. Someone who requested me by name. Someone who trusts me with their image.

I cut his hair. We talk. We laugh. We connect. It's not just a transaction. It's a relationship. It's art. It's service. It's both of us leaving better than we came.

Throughout the day, I have clients like that. People who appreciate the craft. People who value quality. People who don't rush me. People who let me do my best work.

Around 1 PM, I take a break. Not because I have to. But because I can. Because I own the shop. I make the schedule. I listen to my body. And when my body says rest, I rest.

I eat lunch. Something I cooked. Something healthy. Something that helps my lupus instead of hurting it. And I enjoy it. No rushing. No stressing. Just enjoying food.

By 2 PM, I'm back to cutting. More clients. More conversations. More art. More service.

At 5 PM, my last client leaves. And I clean up my station. Count my money. And I've made enough. Not just to survive. But to thrive. To save. To invest. To build toward that restaurant. To keep pursuing those acting and modeling dreams.

And then I go home. And I cook dinner. And I work out. Not like I used to. But enough. Enough to stay strong. Enough to keep lupus in check. Enough to feel like I'm still fighting.

And then I rest. Watch TV. Spend time with family. And I go to bed grateful. Grateful I woke up feeling good. Grateful I had a productive day. Grateful I'm building something. Grateful I'm still chasing dreams. Grateful I'm still here.

That's my perfect day. Reasonable. Achievable. But still ambitious. Still dreaming. Still reaching. Just adjusted for the reality of lupus. Just adapted for the body I have now instead of the body I had then.

Well, one of the dreams I gained since lupus that I didn't have before is to be able to do things for my grandkids and maintain a relationship. And to have professional skills in haircutting and cooking.

Before lupus, I was too focused on boxing. Too focused on becoming a champion. Too focused on me. My career. My dreams. My success.

I didn't think about legacy beyond the boxing ring. I didn't think about family beyond making my mom proud. I didn't think about the future beyond the next fight.

But lupus forced me to slow down. Forced me to think bigger. Longer. Deeper.

Now I think about my grandkids. About being there for them. About teaching them. About passing down skills. About showing them how to cook. How to cut hair. How to handle money. How to chase dreams. How to adapt when life knocks you down.

Now I think about relationships. About maintaining them. About investing in them. About being present. About being available. About being the person people can count on. Not just when I'm winning. But always.

Now I think about skills. About mastering crafts. About being professional. About being excellent. Not for fame. Not for money. But for pride. For satisfaction. For the joy of doing something well.

Those are dreams I didn't have before lupus. Or maybe I had them but they were buried under the bigger, louder dream of boxing glory.

But lupus stripped away the noise. Stripped away the distractions. And what's left is what really matters: family, relationships, skills, legacy.

Funny how losing a dream can help you find better ones. Funny how tragedy can lead to clarity. Funny how the worst thing that ever happened to you can also be the thing that saves you.

Not funny ha-ha. Funny strange. Funny ironic. Funny in that way where you look back years later and realize: maybe it all happened exactly the way it was supposed to. Maybe losing boxing was the only way to find everything else. Maybe Pretty Boy the boxer had to die so Johnny the barber, the cook, the grandfather, the survivor could be born.

I don't know if I believe that. I don't know if everything happens for a reason. But I know this: I'm here. I'm still dreaming. I'm still fighting. Just for different things now. And that's okay. That's enough. That's more than enough.

And what dreams really mean, well, I'll tell you.

Dreams aren't about the specific goal. They're about the feeling you think achieving that goal will give you.

I didn't really want to be a professional boxer. I wanted to feel successful. Accomplished. Proud. Respected. Valuable. Like I mattered. Like I wasn't just another kid from Paterson. Like I was somebody.

And when boxing was taken away, I thought those feelings were taken too. But they weren't. Because those feelings don't come from boxing. They come from doing something well. From helping people. From building something. From showing up. From trying. From refusing to quit.

And I can get those feelings from barbering. From cooking. From being a grandfather. From surviving lupus. From writing this book. From helping someone who's struggling. From sharing my story.

The dream changed. But the feeling stayed. And the feeling is what matters.

So to anyone reading this who's lost a dream: the dream might be gone. But the feeling you were chasing? That's still available. You just have to find a new path to it. A different vehicle. An adapted goal.

For me, it was boxing to barbering to cooking to modeling to acting to grandfathering to writing. All different. All leading to the same place: feeling like I matter. Like I'm valuable. Like I'm somebody.

And I am somebody. Not because I'm a boxer. But because I'm a survivor. A fighter. A dreamer. A person who refuses to let circumstances define him. A person who keeps adapting. Keeps trying. Keeps chasing.

That's who I am. That's who lupus forced me to become. That's who I'm proud to be. A decent human being.

Some people think it's sad. "He's still chasing dreams at his age. With his health. He should just accept reality."

But I think it's beautiful. I think it's brave. I think it's necessary.

Because what's the alternative? Stop dreaming? Stop trying? Stop believing things can get better? Stop believing I can achieve something? Stop believing I matter?

No. Not me. Not ever.

I'll chase dreams until I can't chase anymore. And then I'll walk after them. And then I'll crawl. And when I can't crawl, I'll reach. And when I can't reach, I'll dream. Because dreaming is free. Dreaming doesn't require a healthy body. Dreaming just requires hope. And I've got plenty of that.

So yes, I'm signed with Maps Models. Yes, I'm submitting to casting calls. Yes, I'm building my portfolio. Yes,

I'm trying to get on Netflix. Yes, I'm still working toward opening a restaurant. Yes, I'm still perfecting my cuts. Yes, I'm still cooking. Yes, I'm still believing.

Because that's what dreamers do. We dream. Even when it doesn't make sense. Even when the odds are against us. Even when everyone says it's impossible. We dream. We try. We fail. We adjust. We try again.

And maybe I'll make it. Maybe I'll get that Netflix role. Maybe I'll open that restaurant. Maybe I'll cut a famous actor's hair. Maybe I'll be on a commercial. Maybe.

Or maybe I won't. Maybe none of it happens. Maybe I keep grinding and nothing breaks through.

But you know what? I'll still be proud. Because I tried. Because I didn't give up. Because I kept dreaming. Because I refused to let lupus kill my spirit. Because I showed my grandkids: this is what a fighter looks like. Not someone who never loses. But someone who never quits.

That's the real dream. Not success. But persistence. Not winning. But refusing to lose. Not achieving everything. But trying for everything.

And that dream? That dream I'm already living. That dream lupus can't take. That dream is mine forever.

So when people ask me: "What do you do?"

I don't say: "I used to be a boxer."

I say: "I'm a master barber. I cook professionally. I model. I'm trying to break into acting. I'm a grandfather. I'm a lupus survivor. I'm a writer. I'm a dreamer."

All of that. Not one thing. All of it. Because that's who lupus forced me to become. Not limited. But expanded. Not less. But more. Not a failed boxer. But a successful human being.

And you know what? I like this version of me better. He's more interesting. More dimensional. More real. More human.

Pretty Boy was a character. Johnny is a person. And persons are always more valuable than characters. Because characters are one-dimensional. But persons? Persons are infinite. Persons are complex. Persons are deep.

So thank you, lupus. I never thought I'd say that. But thank you. For forcing me to become more than I ever would have been. For forcing me to dream bigger than one boxing ring. For forcing me to see myself as more than fists and footwork.

I'm still Pretty Boy. But now I'm also so much more. And that's the best dream of all. The dream of becoming fully yourself. Completely yourself. Authentically yourself. Not who you thought you should be. But who you actually are.

That's my lupus. That's my problem. That's my dream. And I'm living it every single day.

Chapter 14
How I Spiritually Nourish My Soul

From my prayers to gospel music to traveling through many churches listening to all different types of preachers preach in so many different styles. And how I took an important message that they preached that day with me. And I held on to it in my mind forever.

So yes, when I mean I wanted to give my soul some nourishing and uplifting, I wake up to Donnie McClurkin's gospel show and listen to some inspirational gospel music.

I also take time out to listen to Steve Harvey's radio music show and listen to Steve say the Daily Bread, prayers of the day.

It helps me a lot to be reminded that the power of God helps me get up in the morning. To start my day. And every walk and way in my life.

Your soul needs food just like your body does. You can't just feed your body and starve your soul. That's what I learned. That's what lupus taught me. When your body is failing, your soul better be strong. Because if both fail at the same time, you're done. You're finished. You give up.

So I feed my soul. Every single day. With prayers. With gospel music. With sermons. With scripture. With God's presence. That's how I survive. Not just the meds. Not just the doctors. But the spiritual nourishment. The soul food that keeps me going when everything else wants to quit.

My morning routine now these days when I get up is to get up early and listen to the news and gospel music at the same time.

I know it's weird. But I've been doing that for some years now.

I lay out my meds and start fixing myself breakfast. And then I work out. And then I write my plans down in my notepad for that day.

I look and check on what my plans were for today and the rest of the week. I then check my refrigerator to see what I need to get fresh. I check my bathroom and other house supplies.

And then I am out of the house by 8 AM. And start my missions of the day. And that is my routine every day.

Let me break it down in more detail because my morning routine is sacred to me. It's what keeps me alive. It's what keeps me sane. It's what keeps me believing.

I wake up. Not because I want to. But because my body wakes up. Pain wakes me up. Or stiffness. Or just the habit of years of waking up early. I don't fight it anymore. I just get up.

First thing I do is turn on the TV. News on one channel. And gospel music on my phone. Both at the same time. People think that's weird. How can you listen to two things at once? But I can. The news keeps me connected to the world. Reminds me that life is still happening outside my body. Outside my pain. And the gospel music? That feeds my soul. That reminds me God is still here. Still watching. Still caring.

I go to the kitchen. Lay out my meds. All of them. Line them up. Count them. Make sure I have everything. Prednisone. Plaquenil. Pain meds. Supplements. Water. Orange juice to help them go down. This is my reality. Every morning. A pharmacy on my kitchen counter.

I start making breakfast. Nothing heavy. Usually oatmeal. Or eggs. Or a smoothie. Something light but nutritious. Something that will help the meds work. Something that won't upset my stomach. Because some of these meds are harsh. They need food. They need cushioning.

I take my meds. All of them. One by one. With water. With orange juice. And I pray over them. "God, let these meds work. Let them help. Let them not hurt me. Let them do what they're supposed to do." Every morning. The same prayer. Over pills.

I work out. Not like I used to. Not seven hundred and fifty pullups. Not three-hour runs. But enough. Stretching. Light weights. Exercise bike. Maybe some pushups. Maybe some squats. Whatever my body can handle that day. Some days it's a lot. Some days it's barely anything. But I do something. Because movement is life. And if I stop moving, I start dying.

I shower. Get dressed. And then I sit down with my notepad. My planning notepad. And I write. What am I doing today? What are my missions? What needs to get done? Groceries? Doctor appointment? Barbershop? Cooking? I write it all down. Because if I don't write it down, I forget. Lupus fog. Medication fog. Whatever you want to call it. My memory isn't what it used to be. So I write everything down.

I check my plans for the week. Look at what's coming. Prepare. Anticipate. Adjust if needed. Then I check the refrigerator. What do I need to get fresh? What's running low? What expired? Then I check the bathroom. Toilet paper? Soap? Towels? Then other house supplies. Cleaning products? Laundry detergent? Everything.

I'm out of the house. Missions begin. Errands. Appointments. Work. Whatever the day requires. And I'm ready. Because I prepared. Because I planned. Because I fed my soul and my body. Because I'm not just surviving. I'm living.

That's my routine. Every single day. Has been for years. It's what keeps me going. It's what gives me structure. It's what reminds me I'm still here. Still fighting. Still believing.

Well, what specific gospel songs I listen to in the morning that actually speak to me spiritually?

Well, I listen to an artist by the name of Kirk Franklin. "1-2-3 Victory." He sings the song that celebrates what God has done and will continue to do.

I listen to the artist Jonathan McReynolds. He sings a song about finding relief from life's pressure by turning to the Lord.

And songs like "Never Would Have Made It" by Marvin Sapp.

I listen to Kirk Franklin again because I like his other songs. Like "My Life Is in Your Hands." "Bless Me." "A God Like You." "Help Me Believe." And "Wanna Be Happy."

So yes, those are a few of the gospel songs that definitely make me happy and speak to me spiritually.

But let me tell you why these songs specifically. Because it's not random. It's not just because they sound good. It's because they speak to my situation. They speak to my pain. They speak to my struggle.

"1-2-3 Victory" by Kirk Franklin: That song is about celebrating what God has already done. Not what He's going to do. Not what you hope He'll do. But what He's already done. And when I listen to that song, I remember: I'm still here. I survived that operation when I was nineteen. I survived the diagnosis. I survived the flares. I survived the hospital stays. I survived the moments I wanted to give up. God already gave me victory. I'm living in it right now. That's why I celebrate. Not because

life is easy. But because I'm still here despite lupus trying to kill me.

"Never Would Have Made It" by Marvin Sapp: That's
my anthem. That's the song that speaks directly to me.
Because it's true. I never would have made it without
God. Never. The lyrics say it all: I'm stronger, I'm wiser,
I'm better, much better. That's me. That's my testimony. Without God, I would have given up years ago.
But with God? I'm stronger than lupus. I'm wiser than
the disease. I'm better than my circumstances. That
song reminds me of that every single morning.

Jonathan McReynolds about finding relief from life's
pressure: Life with lupus is pressure. Constant pressure. Physical pressure. Financial pressure. Emotional
pressure. Mental pressure. And sometimes it feels like
you're going to break. Like you can't handle one more
thing. And that's when I turn to the Lord. That's when
I pray. That's when I listen to that song and remember:
I don't have to carry this alone. God carries it with me.
He takes some of the weight. He gives me relief. Not
always physical relief. But spiritual relief. Peace in the
storm. Strength in the struggle.

Kirk Franklin's other songs: "My Life Is in Your Hands"
reminds me I'm not in control. Lupus isn't in control.
God is in control. "Bless Me" is my prayer every morning. God, bless me today. Let me make it through. Let
me be productive. Let me help someone. "A God Like
You" reminds me there's nobody like my God. No doctor. No medicine. No person. Only God. "Help Me Believe" is for the days when doubt creeps in. When pain

makes me question. When fear makes me wonder. God, help me believe. Even when it's hard. Especially when it's hard. "Wanna Be Happy" is simple. It's honest. I want to be happy. Despite lupus. Despite pain. Despite everything. I still want to be happy. And God wants that for me too.

These songs aren't just music. They're medicine. They're therapy. They're survival tools. They're what I reach for when meds aren't enough. When doctors can't help. When nothing else works. These songs remind me: God is still here. God is still working. God is still fighting for me.

A specific message I hear from a sermon is Marvin Sapp. How his song "Never Would Have Made It" comes on when I am feeling down and depressed.

It's like he's telling me: You have to fight and keep on fighting. To want to live and do better with yourself and your life living with lupus.

But let me expand on that. Because it's more than just a song. It's a message from God through Marvin Sapp.

There was this one time I was really down. Really depressed. Really ready to give up. I was in so much pain. The lupus was active. My joints were on fire. My face was swollen. My legs were bleeding from the open sores. I was lying in bed thinking: What's the point? Why keep fighting? Why keep going through this?

And right at that moment, "Never Would Have Made It" came on. Not on the radio. Not on TV. But in my head. I wasn't even listening to music. But I heard that song clear as day. Like God was playing it specifically for me. Specifically for that moment.

And the message was clear: You have to fight. You have to keep fighting. Not because it's easy. Not because you feel like it. But because you have to. Because giving up isn't an option. Because your life matters. Because your story matters. Because someone else needs to hear how you made it through. So they can make it through too.

That message changed my perspective. Because up until that moment, I was fighting for me. To survive. To make it another day. But after that message? I realized I'm not just fighting for me. I'm fighting for my grandkids. For my fiancée. For my family. For everyone who's watching. For everyone who's struggling with their own battles. I'm fighting so they can see: it's possible. You can make it. You can survive. You can live with lupus and still have joy. Still have purpose. Still have meaning.

That message from Marvin Sapp through that song on that particular day? That saved my life. That kept me going. That reminded me why I fight. Not just to survive. But to thrive. To inspire. To prove that lupus doesn't get the final word. God does.

I visited four churches in the past twenty years. Two in Paterson, New Jersey. And two in NYC. One in Harlem and one in the Bronx.

I can't say which one is my favorite. It doesn't feel right. Because each one holds someone special inside of each of the churches. That I like to see either preach the Word of God or a church member who gives powerful testimonials.

Let me tell you about each one:

Church One in Paterson: This was a small church. A storefront church. Nothing fancy. But the pastor there? He was real. He was authentic. He didn't preach prosperity gospel. He preached struggle gospel. He preached survival gospel. He talked about pain. About suffering. About how God doesn't always take away the problem but gives you strength to deal with it. That resonated with me. Because that's my life. God didn't take away lupus. But He gave me strength to live with it.

Church Two in Paterson: This was bigger. More traditional. Beautiful building. Great choir. But what I loved most was this one church member. An older woman. Must have been in her 80s. And every testimony service, she'd get up. And she'd talk about her struggles. Her health issues. Her financial problems. Her family drama. But then she'd always end with: "But God is still good." Every single time. No matter how bad her week was. "But God is still good." That taught me something. Gratitude isn't about your circumstances. It's about your perspective.

Church in Harlem: This church was powerful. The energy. The worship. The preaching. It was like being in the presence of God Himself. The pastor there preached about not letting your circumstances define you. About being more than your diagnosis. About being more than your pain. That message hit me hard. Because I was letting lupus define me. I was "Johnny with lupus." But after that sermon? I'm Johnny. Who happens to have lupus. But lupus doesn't have me.

Church in the Bronx: This church was multicultural. People from everywhere. Different languages. Different cultures. But all worshipping the same God. And there was this one preacher there who talked about how God uses broken people. How God doesn't just use the strong. He uses the weak. The sick. The struggling. Because that's when His power shows up best. That gave me purpose. I'm not broken despite lupus. I'm useful because of lupus. God can use my story. God can use my struggle. God can use my pain to help someone else.

So which is my favorite? I can't choose. Each one gave me something I needed. Each one fed my soul in different ways. Each one reminded me: you're not alone. God is with you. And His people are with you too.

What were the times I felt God's presence very strongly? I can't say just one moment. Because I feel His presence so many times. A lot of moments.

But I can pick one of the moments that still stays with me till this day.

When I was nineteen years old, I was diagnosed with abnormal lymph nodes in my belly. On the side of my abdomen area.

So I had to go under emergency surgery. Because of the pain. It was so severe that I couldn't bear it.

So as they put me to sleep and began surgery, they ended up taking out the wrong lymph nodes. They took out lymph nodes from my left side of the abdomen. But it was the right side lymph nodes they were looking for. They were looking to see if I had cancer in the lymph nodes. But ended up finding nothing. Everything was okay.

See, the second time they did the surgery for the right side of the lymph nodes, it must have been too much for me and my body.

They did both surgeries in four days. So that's like back to back, in a way.

So they actually lost me on the operating table for about ten to fifteen seconds. Maybe more. Can't quite remember exactly.

So that is probably one of the strongest presences of God I felt from Him.

Let me explain. And please bear with me. Because this is hard to talk about. But it's important. Because it's the moment I knew without a doubt that God is real. That heaven is real. That there's something beyond this life.

The time I believe they said they lost me on the operation table had to be when I saw the light.

Yes, it's true. You do get to see the light.

And I also saw my life repeating itself. It was as if my life was going backwards.

Example: The whole time I was in the hospital, from the first day being admitted to the time my family was coming to visit me until the operation was over with to the second operation. I saw the first person who came to visit me to the last. But it started with the last person first to the first person last.

And I just kept saying to myself: "Hey, I saw all of you already. Why are y'all keep coming to visit back and forth like you never left?"

And I just rolled my eyes all the way up. Looking back into the light.

And then I saw all these real tall shadows standing around my bed. And they all were doing a lot of mumbling. Couldn't hear or figure out what they were saying.

But one of the shadows grabbed my hand and said, "Hi, Johnny. How are you?"

I said, "I am okay."

Then it said, "Did you think you were alive the whole time people were coming here to see you?"

I said, "Yeah. My mom and brothers and sister."

And then another one of the shadows said: "You were not alive when all those people were coming to see you. You were dead the whole entire time."

I was like in shock. Like, "No, no, no."

So then another shadow started talking. And it said, "Well, now you know you're dead. What do you want to do?"

I said, "I want to live. Please. I have a baby daughter I have to take care of. And my mother and family need me."

So then a powerful voice out of all the voices of the tall shadows was so loud my body trembled really hard. And it said, "Well, if you want to live, come on. Come on. Come back home."

And I opened my eyes. And started to see clearly who was all there. I was in a surgical room hooked up to many machines to keep me breathing.

And yes, this is all before I had lupus.

I tell you, I still get the chills. And still have dreams of that day and time. Thirty-four years later.

Yes, this all took place when I was nineteen years old. That's when I knew there was a God. And I felt God's presence.

That experience changed everything for me. Because before that, I believed in God kind of casually. Like most people. I went to church sometimes. I prayed sometimes. But I didn't really know if God was real. If heaven was real. If there was anything beyond this life.

But after that? I know. I don't believe. I know. I saw it. I experienced it. I was dead. And God brought me back. Not because I deserved it. Not because I earned it. But because He wasn't done with me yet. Because I had a daughter who needed me. Because my family needed me. Because He had a purpose for my life that wasn't finished yet.

And that knowledge? That certainty? That's what gets me through lupus. Because I know this life isn't all there is. I know there's something beyond this pain. Beyond this struggle. Beyond this body that's failing me. And I know God is with me. Every step. Every day. Every moment. Because He's already proven it. He already brought me back once. And He'll keep me here as long as He needs me here.

So you ask: What does prayer look like for me? And do I have a specific prayer I say daily?

Yes. Every night I say:

"Dear God, bless my whole family. God, bless my mother and father's side. God, bless my fiancée and her friends and family. God, please bless my daughter and my grandkids and family.

God, please bless my surroundings. Please bless Your angels who watch over me. Bless Your animals and creatures of the earth.

God, bless all Your children with special needs. And that were born with a special gift like lupus and any other disease that can relate to the similar illness we have to put up with and deal with for our natural lives You blessed us to be here on Earth.

God, thank You for everything You have been doing for me from birth. Thank You, God, for keeping me here on Earth to experience life itself with loved ones and others from Your kingdom.

God, I love You with all my heart. Amen."

That is my daily prayer.

I say this prayer every single night. Without fail. No matter how tired I am. No matter how much pain I'm in. No matter what kind of day I had. I say this prayer. Because it grounds me. It reminds me what's important. It connects me to God. It connects me to everyone I love. It connects me to everyone who's struggling like me.

And notice what I pray for: Not myself. Not my health. Not my pain. I pray for everyone else first. My family. My fiancée. My daughter. My grandkids. My surroundings. The angels. The animals. All of God's children with special needs and chronic illness. Everyone before me.

Because I learned something: When you pray for others, God takes care of you. When you put others first, God doesn't forget you. When you focus on blessing others, God blesses you. That's how it works. That's the principle. That's the promise.

And at the end, I thank God. Not for taking away lupus. Not for healing me. But for keeping me here. For letting me experience life. For giving me loved ones. For letting me be part of His kingdom. For everything He's been doing since birth. Not just the good things. But everything. Because even the hard things? Even the painful things? Even lupus? It's all part of His plan. It's all shaping me. It's all making me who I'm supposed to be.

How do I maintain my faith when in severe pain?

Because every time I am in pain, I pray.

And when I pray, God's presence will enter my home and let me know He's here by my side. Because I am always feeling a warmish feeling throughout my body. Like God was rubbing His hands across my head and saying a prayer to cast away the pain in my body.

And I tell you, it is so real that this happens most of the times I pray. Right away. Not wasting time looking to take medications before giving God a try and a chance to use His healing power.

And just to witness this all the time is why I keep my faith in myself and God that I'll be alright.

Let me be clear about something: I'm not saying don't take your meds. I'm not saying God replaces medicine. I take my meds. I go to my doctors. I follow medical advice. But I also pray. Because God works through medicine. God works through doctors. But God also works directly. Supernaturally. Miraculously.

And I've experienced it too many times to deny it. I'll be in severe pain. My joints on fire. My body aching. My head pounding. And I'll pray. And I'll feel it. A warmth. Starting at the top of my head. Spreading down through my body. Like God's hands are literally on me. Literally touching me. Literally healing me.

And the pain doesn't always go away completely. But it lessens. It becomes bearable. It becomes manageable. And I feel peace. Not just physical relief. But spiritual peace. The peace that says: You're going to be okay. I'm here with you. You're not alone.

That's how I maintain my faith in severe pain. Not by denying the pain. Not by pretending it doesn't exist. But by inviting God into the pain. By letting Him sit with me in it. By trusting that He's using it for something. By believing that even in the pain, He's still good. He's still faithful. He's still here.

Has my relationship with God ever wavered? And what brought me back?

Well, there have been times years ago when I first started to learn how to deal with lupus. That affected me on how I could believe that God is watching over me.

Because when I was going back and forth to the hospitals because varicose veins were popping out of my legs causing me to bleed very heavily in so many public places. Causing people to look at me like: "Wow, what is going on with him?"

It was times when my arthritis would be so active in the early mornings and I couldn't get out of bed right away.

It was times I was in the doctor's office and the doctors didn't understand lupus. And they treated me like I was an alien from space carrying many diseases that would spread to them if they touched me.

Especially when they would question me about the rashes on my face, my arms, and legs. While I am suffering with so much pain, all they want to do is take turns with different nurses looking at my body parts. Frowning their faces up at me like: "Ewww, I don't want to touch him. What's he got going on with himself?"

So it was like in so many ways: "Please go somewhere else." Basically, they didn't want to be bothered.

It was times I was in search to find a good doctor. And I entered a facility and went to sign my name at the receptionist's desk. The receptionist showed me that they don't want to deal with people of color.

I remember asking a receptionist for a pen to sign my name on the waiting list. And the receptionist threw the pen, making it hit the floor. And once I picked it up and signed my name and then she asked for my insurance card, the receptionist put on rubber gloves and got a paper napkin and told me, "Just put it on here and step back. Or go sit down." Not even saying thank you or "you can have a seat."

So as I waited for an hour and a half, the receptionist told me the doctor didn't accept my insurance.

I told the receptionist, "But my insurance provider told me this doctor does accept my insurance. That's why I am here."

The receptionist kept telling me, "Well, he doesn't. Have a nice day. Please, can you leave?"

I was so in shock. I was so angry. That I started to question God in my prayers.

By saying: "God, why are You letting me go through this? Why are You letting this happen to me? I am doing everything I am supposed to do that is good for myself. I am doing everything I am supposed to do by You."

I started wondering: Is there even a God?

And right away, God brought back memories about what I'd been through when they lost me on the operation table in the year of 1997.

And I said, "I almost forgot where I came from. God, please forgive me. Please, please, please."

And I was brought back to God, knowing He still watches over me. And He gave me a message in so many ways letting me know: Finding a good doctor is not going to be easy.

Let me explain what happened in my spirit at that moment. Because it's important.

I was sitting in my car in that parking lot. Crying. Angry. Hurt. Humiliated. Questioning everything. Questioning God. And then suddenly, like a movie playing in my head, I saw it. The operation. The light. The shadows. Being dead. Being told I was dead. Choosing to live. The powerful voice saying, "Come back home." Opening my eyes in that surgical room.

And it hit me: God saved me then. When I was nineteen. He brought me back from death. Why would He do that just to abandon me now? Why would He save me then just to let me suffer now without Him?

And I heard Him speak. Not audibly. But in my spirit. Clear as day: "I didn't bring you back to leave you. I brought you back because I have plans for you. And those plans include lupus. Those plans include this struggle. Those plans include this pain. Because I'm going to use it all. I'm going to use your story. I'm going to use your testimony. I'm going to use your survival to help someone else survive. But you have to trust Me. Even when it doesn't make sense. Even when people are cruel. Even when doctors turn you away. Even when it hurts. You have to trust Me."

And I broke. Not in a bad way. But in a surrendering way. And I said: "God, I'm sorry. I almost forgot. I almost forgot You saved me. I almost forgot You chose me. I almost forgot You have a purpose for my life. Please forgive me. I trust You. Even through this. Even through the racism. Even through the pain. Even through the rejection. I trust You."

And from that moment, my relationship with God was restored. Stronger than before. Because I remembered: He already proved Himself. He already showed up. He already saved me. So I can trust Him now. In this. In lupus. In all of everything that is happening to me.

So you ask me: What role does my fiancée play in my spiritual life?

Oh, well, let me tell you. Wow. She is the biggest reason why I can understand and truly, truly believe in God. If I ever have doubts, it wasn't me. Trust me when I tell you this.

Every second. Every minute. Every hour. Every day and night. My fiancée will make sure I pray for everything I do. Everything someone does for me.

She makes sure we pray for every move we make together. Pray for every move we make alone.

She makes sure we pray for a good parking space when coming home after we finished running our errands.

She makes sure we bless the food before I cook the food. Bless that the food comes out the way it looks. Yes, she has jokes.

We can go in a shoe store, try out a pair of shoes, and she will say to me: "Oh, God, bless us we don't have stink feet."

I look at her and say to myself: "She's unbelievable. Oh my God." But I love her.

So you tell me: What do you think about how she plays a part in my spiritual life?

My fiancée is my spiritual accountability partner. My prayer warrior. My reminder that God is in everything. Not just the big things. But the small things too. The parking spaces. The food. The shoes. Everything.

Before I met her, I prayed. But not like this. I prayed when things were bad. When I was in pain. When I needed something. But she taught me: pray always. Pray for everything. Pray without ceasing. Not just when you're desperate. But when you're grateful. When you're happy. When you're blessed. When you're just living life.

She taught me that prayer isn't just about asking. It's about acknowledging. Acknowledging that God is in control. That God is present. That God is involved in every detail of your life. Even the parking spaces. Even the food. Even making sure your feet don't stink when you try on shoes at the store.

And at first, I thought it was too much. Too extreme. Too religious. But then I realized: she's right. Because when you pray for everything, you start seeing God in everything. You start noticing His blessings. His provision. His presence. You start living in constant communion with Him. Not just on Sundays. Not just when you're in trouble. But always. Every moment. Every decision. Every breath.

That's what my fiancée gave me. A constant awareness of God. A constant connection to Him. A constant gratitude for Him. And that's changed everything. Now I don't just survive lupus. I survive it with God. Every second. Every minute. Every hour. Every day. Every night.

So how do I share my faith with others who are struggling?

I tell them my life story.

I give them some of a story that just happened recently to me. And how God blessed me because I kept my faith strong in Him.

For example, I told a friend who was homeless and was suffering with diabetes really bad. He wanted to get out of the shelter and get into an apartment. And he wanted a part-time job to get back on his feet.

So I told him I was in a similar situation. Just I was living with my mom. But I had no job. I had no driver's license. I had no income coming in on my side to help my mom. I could barely get around because of my varicose veins in my legs. And the lupus just wouldn't ease up. So I couldn't be outside in scorching heat and sun.

So on my spare time that I had with myself, I would try to get a better relationship with God so He could point me or lead me in the right path of my life. So I prayed.

And I prayed hard every day. I read the Bible and studied the scriptures like I was in a contest of mastering it by heart.

And the more I did this, I felt God's presence. So I knew He was listening to my prayers.

Every time I was alone doing heavy thinking about what I am going to do with my life, it was like I could hear God's voice in my head.

It's like He was talking to me spiritually. All the time I made a move. All the time I was feeling depressed. Every time when it looked like I wanted to give up on myself.

It's like God was telling me so often:

"It will get harder before it gets better. Once it gets better for you, you will know how to appreciate your life more. You won't take anything for granted.

But you've got to keep fighting for a better you. Everybody knows something good like a life on the sunny side doesn't come easy.

You have to first keep that faith strong in believing your God's got your back no matter what. You also must believe in yourself on top of everything else.

No matter what's going on with your situation, everyone gets a setback at some time or at some point in life. That's just God letting you know: No one is perfect or exempt from failure at some point in time.

No one can be on top forever. When you get these set-backs, it's to remind you that God can give it all to you and God can take it all from you. Especially when you're not counting your blessings. Believe that. It happened to me so many times."

And that's how I share my faith to a person who's struggling.

I told my homeless friend with diabetes exactly what God told me. Word for word. And I told him: "This is what got me through. This is what kept me going. This is what changed my life. Not denying the struggle. Not pretending it's easy. But trusting God in the middle of it. Believing He's going to use it. Believing He's going to make something good come from it. Believing it will get better. Not immediately. But eventually. If you keep fighting. If you keep believing. If you keep trusting."

And my friend listened. And he cried. And he said: "I needed to hear that. I needed to know I'm not alone. I needed to know someone else made it through. Because if you made it, maybe I can make it too."

And that's how faith is shared. Not by preaching. Not by judging. Not by quoting scripture at people. But by sharing your story. By being honest about your struggle. By admitting you wanted to give up but didn't. By showing them: if God brought me through, He can bring you through too. You're not alone. God's got your back. And I've got your back. And together, we'll make it.

I also had to recognize: Anything you're trying to do good in your life, it's not going to be easy. Nor a walk in the park. It will be a lot of unexpected challenges. Especially with close family and friends.

Because most of the time, the people who will try to turn your dreams down is someone who knows you a lot more than a stranger you're telling about your plans for the better of your lifestyle.

I myself had to get very disciplined in not telling anyone about my plans unless the person's involved in my plans.

One thing I did learn during my life journey is: Mostly the closest family and friends that envy you, you will never really know it until you tell them or show them about what you're working on for yourself.

And a few months later, because they were in a better position to get your idea faster than you, they take your ideas and maybe switch it up a bit. You know, put a spin on it. Hope that you don't recognize it. And then try to throw it up in your face.

So now that you've seen this so-called good family member or friend steal your idea, you have to go back to your lab and rethink something you can do to earn a better living for yourself. And God knows it's not easy.

But here's what I learned spiritually from that: People will disappoint you. Family will betray you. Friends will steal from you. But God never will. People's support is conditional. But God's support is unconditional. People will turn on you. But God never turns on you.

So I stopped putting my faith in people. I put my faith in God. I stopped sharing my dreams with everyone. I share them with God first. And if He blesses them, if He opens doors, if He makes a way, then I know it's right. And if people steal my ideas? God will give me better ones. If people betray me? God will send better people. If people turn on me? God never will.

That's the spiritual lesson lupus taught me. Not to trust in people. But to trust in God. Not to rely on human strength. But to rely on divine strength. Not to seek approval from others. But to seek approval from God. Because at the end of the day, people will fail you. But God never fails you.

So how do I nourish my soul spiritually for my own fulfillment?

I wake up with gospel music and news. I pray over my meds. I pray over my breakfast. I pray over my plans. I listen to Kirk Franklin, Marvin Sapp, Jonathan McReynolds. I remember sermons that changed my perspective. I remember churches that fed my soul. I remember that moment at 19 when God brought me back from death. I pray my daily prayer for everyone I love. I invite God into my pain. I remember He's never abandoned me. I let my fiancée remind me to pray for everything. And I share my faith with others who are struggling.

That's how I nourish my soul. Not once a week on Sunday. But every single day. Every single moment. Because my soul needs constant nourishment. Just like my body needs constant medication. My soul needs constant connection to God.

And that's how I survive. Not just physically. But spiritually. Not just with a body that's still breathing. But with a soul that's still thriving. Still believing. Still trusting. Still worshipping. Still grateful. Still connected to God.

That's my lupus. That's my problem. That's my solution. God. Always God. Forever God. No matter what.

Chapter 15
Did God Bless Me with Lupus to Make Me A Wiser Person?

Well, let me start by saying that growing up in my early teenage years, I was told by my mom and the rest of my siblings and associates that I made some wrong choices in life. On things I wanted to do in life. On who I was spending it with. At the time, to put it simply, I hung out with the wrong crowd of friends.

When I was younger in my teenager years, the types of crowds I hung around did not have a good example of role models. Most of the guys either smoked cigarettes or pot. And did some sort of drinking liquor beverages.

They loved hanging out in clubs that were full of violence. They loved to hang in violence and drug-infested areas. They even drove cars without proper paperwork.

They also liked starting trouble in the streets with others that were into the same thing they were into. Because they wanted the biggest name in the neighborhood streets to the hometown.

So yes, the crowd I hung out with was not too good. With me or my mother. She didn't approve of it.

Let me be more specific about who these guys were and what we were doing. Because "wrong crowd" doesn't tell the full story. And if I'm being honest, I need to own what I was part of.

These weren't just guys who made bad choices. These were guys who lived bad choices. Who embraced bad choices. Who took pride in bad choices.

They smoked cigarettes like chimneys. Pack after pack. Everywhere. In cars. In basements. On street corners. Walking down the block. Didn't matter. Always smoking.

And pot? That was daily. Multiple times a day. Wake and bake in the morning. Smoke during the day. Smoke at night. Some of them couldn't function without it. Some of them wouldn't function without it.

The drinking was constant. Not social drinking. Not casual drinking. But heavy drinking. Liquor. Vodka. Hennessy. Whatever they could get. However they could get it. Whether they were old enough or not. Whether they had money or not. They found a way.

And the clubs? These weren't nice clubs. These weren't family clubs. These were clubs where fights broke out every weekend. Where people got stabbed. Where people got shot. Where violence was expected. Where violence was normal. And these guys? They loved it. They fed off it. They looked for it.

They hung out in the worst neighborhoods. The drug corners. The trap houses. The places where dealers worked. Where addicts came. Where cops raided. They weren't just passing through. They were planted there. Part of the scene. Part of the problem.

And the cars? They'd drive without licenses. Without insurance. Without registration. Stolen plates. Expired inspection. Didn't matter. They'd drive anyway. And when they got pulled over? They'd run. Or lie. Or have someone else take the charge.

But the worst part? The violence they started. The fights they picked. The beefs they created. All for reputation. All for respect. All to have the biggest name in the streets. That's what mattered to them. Not family. Not future. Not life. Just street reputation. Just being known. Just being feared.

And my mother? She saw it all. She knew who these guys were. She knew what they were doing. She knew what I was becoming. And she didn't approve. Not one bit. She'd tell me: "Johnny, those boys are going to get you killed. Or locked up. Or worse. You need to leave them alone. You need to find better friends. You need to choose better."

But I didn't listen. I thought I knew better. I thought I was different. I thought I could handle it. I was wrong.

I ended up getting in trouble all the time. But I got away with most of it to the point where I almost thought I was untouchable.

So I started to really believe it. To where it felt normal. Yeah, right. What was I thinking?

What type of trouble did I get into? Well, I got into trouble driving without a license at some point. Being involved with the wrong crowd.

I got kicked out of high school because of playing hooky with the wrong crowd of friends.

I got suspended from fighting in class. Hanging and listening to the wrong group of friends.

Let me tell you about the specific incidents. Because saying "I got in trouble" doesn't capture how stupid I was. How reckless. How close I came to destroying my future.

Driving without a license: I was sixteen. Didn't have my license yet. But my boy had a car. And he was drunk. Too drunk to drive. So I said, "I'll drive." No license. No permit. Just confidence. And stupidity. We got pulled over. Cop asked for license and registration. I had neither. My friend was passed out in the back seat. The cop could have arrested me. Could have impounded the car. Could have called my mom. But he didn't. He gave me a warning. Told me to park the car and walk home. Said, "You're lucky tonight. Don't be stupid again." I was lucky. But did I learn? No. I kept driving without a license. Multiple times. Until I finally got caught for real and had to go to court. That's when my mom lost it. That's when she said, "You're going to end up dead or in jail. And I can't save you from yourself."

Playing hooky and getting kicked out: I wasn't just skipping one class. I was skipping entire days. Weeks. I'd go to school in the morning. Sign in. Then leave with my boys. We'd go to someone's house. Smoke. Drink. Play video games. Do nothing. And I thought I was getting away with it. Until the school called my mom. Told her I'd missed forty days. Forty. In one semester. They said, "Your son is failing everything. He's not coming to class. And when he does come, he's disruptive. He's fighting. He's causing problems. We're recommending expulsion." My mom cried. Not angry crying. Hurt crying. Disappointed crying. She said, "I didn't raise you like this. I didn't struggle for you to throw your life away. What happened to you?"

Fighting in class: There was this one time. Another student said something disrespectful. I don't even remember what. Something small. Something that didn't matter. But I was with my boys. And I had a reputation to protect. So I snapped. Started swinging. Right there in class. Teacher tried to break it up. I pushed the teacher. Not hard. But enough. Security came. Dragged me out. Suspended me for two weeks. And the worst part? My boys thought it was funny. Thought I was tough. Thought I was cool. But my mom? She was humiliated. She had to come to school. Had to meet with the principal. Had to hear about her son acting like a thug. And I saw it in her eyes: shame. I made my mother ashamed of me. That's what I did.

So at the time of me making these wrong choices, and as I started to become a young adult in my 20s, I started noticing a change in my health.

At what age did I notice health issues? Well, I had a couple of health issues growing up. I was a preemie. I was born early. I was born at five months instead of nine months.

So I used to have really bad asthma. I used to get nose-bleeds really bad when I was in too much heat.

So when I turned about 26 years old is when I started to see a different side and different styles of my health issues.

I started noticing my skin being very dry. I started noticing my legs swollen very often. I started noticing my weight loss. My hair loss. I started noticing my face started to be reddish around the eyes, leaving a rash-type look.

I started noticing not having a big appetite for food or urge to eat anything.

I was always catching hot flashes. I started noticing my body was always sore, especially in the morning. I thought it was because I wasn't working out every day like I used to in my teenager years.

But like I said, once I started having these symptoms, I started making appointments to see a doctor.

Let me break down what was happening to my body at 26. Because these weren't small things. These weren't things you could ignore. These were warning signs. Alarm bells. My body screaming: Something is wrong.

My skin: It was so dry it would crack. Bleed. I'd put lotion on. Didn't help. I'd drink water. Didn't help. It was like my skin was dying. Peeling. Flaking. Especially on my hands. My arms. My legs. I looked like I had some kind of disease. People would stare. Ask questions. "What's wrong with your skin?" I didn't know. I had no answer.

My legs: They'd swell up like balloons. Especially at night. I'd take my socks off. The indentations would stay for hours. My ankles would be twice their normal size. It hurt to walk. Hurt to stand. Hurt to move. I thought maybe I was standing too much. Working too much. But it kept happening. Every day. Getting worse.

My weight: I was losing weight without trying. And I was eating. But the weight kept falling off. I went from two hundred and ten pounds to a hundred and eight-five pounds in three months. People said, "You look good. You losing weight?" But I wasn't trying to lose weight. It was just happening. And that scared me.

My hair: It started thinning. Then falling out. In the shower. On my pillow. In my hands. I'd run my fingers through my hair and come away with handfuls. I was too young to be going bald. Way too young. But it was happening anyway.

My face: The redness around my eyes. The butterfly rash. I didn't know what it was at the time. I thought maybe it was an allergic reaction. Or eczema. Or something I ate. But it wouldn't go away. It would get worse. Brighter. More visible. People started asking, "Did you get sunburned?" I hadn't been in the sun. This was something else.

My appetite: Gone. I'd look at food and feel sick. I'd try to eat and couldn't. Nothing tasted good. Nothing looked good. I went from eating three big meals a day to barely eating one small meal. And even that was a struggle. My mom would cook my favorite foods. I'd take two bites and be done. She'd say, "Johnny, you have to eat. You're wasting away." But I couldn't. I had no appetite. No desire. No hunger.

The hot flashes: They'd come out of nowhere. I'd be sitting there, fine. Then suddenly, I'd be drenched in sweat. My shirt soaked. My face dripping. Like I'd just run a marathon. But I was just sitting. Just existing. And it would pass. Then come back. Over and over. All day. All night.

The soreness: Every morning, I'd wake up feeling like I'd been hit by a truck. My whole body ached. My joints hurt. My muscles hurt. My bones hurt. It took me 30 minutes just to get out of bed. To stretch enough to move. To loosen up enough to function. And I thought: Maybe I'm getting old. Maybe this is what happens when you stop working out. But I was only 26. This wasn't normal.

So I started going to doctors. Trying to figure out what was wrong. Trying to get answers. Trying to fix whatever was broken inside me.

To where it would set me back to thinking really hard to myself and saying: "My God, what is going on with me? I eat healthy most of the time and work out daily. Why does my body keep breaking down like it's not paying off with most of the good things I'm doing to keep myself in shape? What am I doing wrong?"

The time I realized God was trying to tell me something was when I couldn't get my health issues on track in the way I wanted.

I was like: "Wow, what is going on with me? Why is this happening to me? Did someone poison me? Did someone put a curse on me?"

"I am going to all these different doctors for all these different symptoms. And nothing seems to be getting better. Do these doctors know what they're doing?"

Then I started thinking, "Damn! Is God trying to tell me something? Is God trying to tell me to change my life around? Is God telling me I need to start paying attention to what I eat? Where at and where from? From someone's house or a restaurant? Should I be cooking my own food I like to eat so I know what's in it? I don't know. I was confused."

Let me tell you about that moment. The exact moment. When everything clicked. When I finally understood that this isn't random. This isn't bad luck. This is God.

I was sitting in yet another doctor's office. Waiting for yet another test result. And the doctor came in with that look. That "I don't know what's wrong with you" look. And he said, "Your labs are abnormal. But we're not sure why. We need to run more tests. Come back in two weeks." And I snapped. Not at him. But inside. In my head. I thought: This is the fifth doctor. The tenth round of tests. The hundredth time hearing "we don't know." Something is seriously wrong. And nobody can tell me what it is. Nobody can fix it. Nobody can help.

And that's when it hit me. Like a voice. Not audible. But clear. In my spirit. In my soul: "Johnny, I'm trying to get your attention. I'm trying to tell you something. You're not listening with your ears. So I'm speaking through your body. Through your pain. Through your symptoms. You need to change. You need to stop. You need to turn around. Before it's too late."

And I sat there in that parking lot after that appointment. And I thought about my life. About the choices I'd made. About the people I'd hung around. About the trouble I'd gotten into. About the lifestyle I was living. And I realized: God didn't cause this. But He's using this. To wake me up. To get my attention. To force me to see what I was doing to myself. To make me choose: Keep going this way and die. Or change and live.

That's when I knew. God was trying to tell me something. And I finally started listening.

So as some of the elders in the family, like uncles and aunts and my mom, always preached to me and reminded me of what I was doing wrong. And started telling me: "This is God trying to give you a sign to start doing the right thing in life and make better choices on who you hang out with and things that you're doing that isn't right."

And she also always said: "You better start praying to God for a more positive mind so you can head on a better path and a future."

And yes, I heard everything my mom and others who I was surrounded by at the time said. But I still wasn't listening nor doing what was said or told.

Until I realized I am really starting to suffer with my health up and down like a roller coaster. One minute I'm doing fine. The next I'm down for the count.

My mom and my elders had been warning me for years. "Johnny, those boys are going to ruin you. Johnny, you need to straighten up. Johnny, God is watching. Johnny, you're going to regret this." And I'd hear them. But I wouldn't listen. I'd nod. Agree. Say, "Yeah, yeah, I know." Then go right back to doing what I was doing.

But now? With my body breaking down? With doctors not having answers? With symptoms multiplying? Their words came back. Haunting me. "This is God trying to give you a sign." And I finally got it. Finally understood. This wasn't punishment. This was intervention. God stepping in. Saying: "Enough. You won't listen to your mom. You won't listen to your elders. So I'm going to speak through your body. Through your pain. Through your health. Until you finally pay attention."

And the message was clear:

"Change your life. Change your friends. Change your choices. Change your path. Or this will kill you. Maybe not today. Maybe not tomorrow. But eventually. You can't keep living like this and expect to survive. Start paying attention to what you eat. Start paying attention to who you're around. Start paying attention to where you go. Start paying attention to what you do. Everything matters now. Everything affects your health. Everything has consequences."

"Pray. Talk to Me. Give Me your time. Give Me your attention. Give Me your life. And I'll guide you. I'll heal you. I'll protect you. But you have to choose Me. You have to choose better. You have to choose life."

That was the message. That's what God was telling me. And this time, I listened.

So I believe this was a starting sign of what was going to make me change my life.

I started saying to myself as I prayed to God, asking Him: "Please, God, help me get right. I don't want to be suffering like this as I get older."

"To see a lot of older elderly, especially my grandparents, who I saw live most of their life in hospitals and doctor's visits."

So I started slowing myself down on everything I do and started to change my life.

But when I prayed really hard to God and started getting close to Him, I almost felt Him talking to me spiritually. Giving me guidance to a positive path to head towards.

And the more I started to believe He was talking to me spiritually, my faith got stronger. And I started feeling healthier and getting back stronger.

I really just couldn't believe it. It almost felt like a miracle because I started feeling really good really quick.

And yes, that is definitely one of the times in life I knew I had to start thinking and living differently for the betterment of myself.

The specific turning point? I can tell you exactly when it happened. Exactly where. Exactly how.

I was at a funeral. Watching them lower the casket into the ground. And I thought about how this person had spent the last years of their life. In and out of hospitals. Doctor's appointments every week. Multiple medications. Pain. Suffering. Barely living. Just existing. And I thought: That's where I'm headed. That's my future. If I don't change. If I don't stop. That's going to be me. Dying slowly. In pain. Regretting everything.

And right then, at that cemetery, I prayed. Not a casual prayer. Not a "bless this food" prayer. But a desperate prayer. A "God, if You're real, I need You now" prayer. I said:

"God, I'm scared. I'm really scared. My body is breaking down. The doctors don't know why. And I'm only twenty-six. I should be in my prime. But I feel like I'm dying. And I know it's my fault. I know I made bad choices. I know I hung with the wrong people. I know I did wrong things. And I'm sorry. I'm really sorry.

Please help me. Please fix me. Please give me another chance. I don't want to die like my grandma. I don't want to spend my life suffering. I want to live. I want to be healthy. I want to do right. I want to make my mom proud. I want to have a family. I want to fulfill my purpose. Please, God. Help me change. Help me heal. Help me live. I'm listening now. I'm ready now. Tell me what to do. And I'll do it. I promise. Just please. Don't let me die like this."

And I felt it. A warmth. A peace. A presence. God was there. Listening. Responding. Not with words. But with a feeling. A knowing. A certainty: "I'm going to help you. But you have to do your part. You have to change. You have to cut off the people who are dragging you down. You have to stop doing things that are killing you. You have to start eating right. Praying right. Living right. And I'll heal you. I'll guide you. I'll protect you. But you have to choose Me. Every day. Every moment. Every decision. Choose Me. And I'll choose you."

That was the turning point. That cemetery. That funeral. That prayer. That moment. Everything changed after that. Everything.

By cutting off the people who don't mean me no good. The food that's not good for me.

And I started educating myself on healing by talking to God spiritually. Giving my time to God whenever I had a chance.

Because I knew I wanted better for myself. Especially if I wanted to live a long, healthy lifestyle.

The changes I made weren't overnight. They were gradual. Step by step. Day by day. But they were real. They were permanent. They were life-saving.

First, I cut off the friends who were bad for me. The guys who smoked. Who drank. Who looked for trouble. Who had no goals. No future. No purpose. I told them: "I can't hang anymore. I'm trying to get my life together. And being around y'all isn't helping." Some understood. Some didn't. But I did it anyway. Because my life depended on it.

Second, I changed my diet. I stopped eating fast food every day. Stopped drinking soda. Stopped eating junk. I started cooking my own meals. Healthy meals. Vegetables. Fruits. Lean meats. Fish. I studied nutrition. Learned what foods help with inflammation. What foods hurt. What my body needed. What it didn't. And I followed it. Strictly. Religiously.

Third, I started praying. Every morning. Every night. Throughout the day. Talking to God. Thanking Him. Asking for guidance. Listening for His voice. And the more I prayed, the clearer things became. The stronger I felt. The more confident I was that I was on the right path.

Fourth, I went back to church. Found a good church. A church that preached truth. That taught the Word. That had people who genuinely cared. And I got involved. Joined a men's group. Started studying the Bible. Started serving. And that community? That support? That accountability? It saved me.

Fifth, I focused on my health. Went to all my doctor's appointments. Took all my meds. Did all my tests. Followed all the instructions. And slowly, gradually, I started feeling better. The symptoms didn't disappear completely. But they improved. And that improvement gave me hope. Gave me motivation. Gave me proof: This is working. God is healing me. I'm on the right path.

And let me tell you how my old friends reacted once they knew I turned my life around for the best of me.

Well, some old friends were so proud of me. And respected me for making a big move like that in my life.

A lot of times they said: "I knew you could do it. This bad lifestyle wasn't for you. You deserved better. I am glad you changed yourself around before you got caught up like we did."

"It's no joke being homeless and can't get help from no one because of a bad reputation from your past."

And some old friends were not too pleasant. They wouldn't even want to spend any time with me or around me.

Once I told them: "I don't hang out no more. I don't be trying to hang with people who are looking for trouble with others anymore."

"I am going back to school. I have a steady girlfriend because I am trying to get married. I want to be married. I want my own family. I just want better for myself."

"And if I can't be around someone who I can't learn nothing positive from, I don't want to be around them."

So they started saying: "So you think you're too good for anyone now?"

I said: "No. Just I want better for myself and my family."

The reactions from my old friends were split. Half were supportive. Half were bitter. And that told me everything I needed to know about who they really were.

The supportive ones? They were guys who secretly wished they could change too. Who saw what was happening to them. Who knew they were going nowhere. Who respected that I had the courage to leave. They'd say things like:

"Yo, Johnny, I'm proud of you, man. For real. You doing the right thing. This street life ain't it. We all know it. But most of us too deep in to get out. You got out early. That's smart. Don't come back. Don't look back. Keep going. Make something of yourself. Show us it's possible."

And some of them? They're still my friends today. From a distance. I'll check on them. See how they're doing. Pray for them. Hope they find their way out too.

But the bitter ones? They took it personally. Like me changing was a judgment on them. Like me wanting better meant I thought I was better. They'd say:

"Oh, so you too good for us now? You think you better than us? You think you're special? You think going to church and getting a girlfriend makes you different? You're still from the same hood. You're still the same dude. Stop acting brand new. Stop acting like you changed. You're going to be right back here. Watch. You're going to fail. And when you do, don't come crying to us."

And you know what? That hurt. Because these were guys I'd known for years. Guys I'd been through things with. Guys I considered brothers. And they couldn't be happy for me. Couldn't support me. Couldn't encourage me. All they could do was hate. Tear down. Try to pull me back. And that showed me: they were never really my friends. They were just people I hung around. People who wanted company in their misery. And when I chose not to be miserable anymore, they couldn't handle it.

So I let them go. No hard feelings. No anger. Just acceptance. We're on different paths now. They chose theirs. I chose mine. And that's okay.

So you ask: What temptations do I face today? And how do I resist?

The temptations I face today are: While driving and someone cuts me off in traffic, I find myself staying angry at the person for a while.

I find myself talking about how stupid the other person was that was driving that other car. Even though it was over with hours ago.

I find myself getting snappy and uptight sometimes with others when I am in pain. It's like I have no patience for anyone when in pain.

When I am out on my journey, I see restaurants I love to eat from. And I know they are expensive.

Each and everything I just mentioned, I resist them by saying a prayer.

I start thinking: "I don't want to be back in that place or time in my life again."

"If I am going to keep moving myself to a better future, I must stay mindful about everything that will be a temptation to put myself backwards in life. With how I was and where I came from."

Let me be real about the temptations. Because they're still there. Every day. Testing me. Challenging me. Trying to pull me back.

Anger in traffic: This one gets me. Someone cuts me off. Doesn't signal. Drives recklessly. And I feel it rising. That old street mentality. That "disrespect has consequences" mindset. And I want to chase them. Follow them. Confront them. Show them they can't do that. But then I catch myself. And I pray. "God, calm me down. It's not worth it. They're not worth it. My health is more important than proving a point. My peace is more valuable than being right." And I let it go. I let them go. I breathe. I move on.

Impatience when in pain: When lupus flares up. When my joints hurt. When my body aches. I become someone else. Short-tempered. Snappy. Rude. My fiancée will ask a simple question. And I'll snap at her. My grandkids will make noise. And I'll yell. And immediately, I regret it. Because they don't deserve that. They're not the enemy. The pain is the enemy. So now, when I feel that irritation rising, I remove myself. I go to another room. I pray. I breathe. I remind myself: "They love you. They're trying to help. Don't push them away because you're hurting. Let them in. Let them support you."

Expensive restaurants: I see them when I'm out. The places I used to love. The food I used to eat. And I'm tempted. So tempted. To just go in. Order what I want. Enjoy it. Live a little. But then I remember: that food will hurt me. Those ingredients will trigger a flare. That one meal isn't worth three days of pain. So I resist. I pray. "God, help me choose what's good for me. Not just what tastes good. But what's actually good for my body. For my health. For my future." And I keep driving. I go home. I cook something healthy. And I feel good about that choice.

Old friends reaching out: Every once in a while, I'll get a call. A text. "Yo, where you been? Come hang out. We miss you." And part of me wants to. Part of me misses them. Misses the old days. The simplicity. The fun. But I know better. I know what "hang out" means. It means drinking. Smoking. Wasting time. Getting into trouble. So I resist. I respond kindly but firmly. "I'm good, bro. Doing my thing. Staying focused. Hope you're well." And I don't engage further. Because I know: one hangout turns into two. Two turns into falling back into old patterns. And I've worked too hard to go backwards.

That's how I resist. Prayer. Remembering where I came from. Remembering where I'm going. Remembering what's at stake. My health. My future. My family. My purpose. It's not always easy. But it's always worth it.

And how can I tell you how lupus made me wiser? For one, and I'm talking for myself, I don't like the idea or the feeling of pain and suffering or being stressed out.

I definitely don't want to keep dealing with having to go back and forth to the hospitals if it can be avoided.

Lupus really made me realize that if you don't start taking life seriously, things with your health can turn for the worse.

And I saw that once I did start to take things with myself in a responsible manner, things started to lighten up for me with my lifestyle and health issues.

Lupus made me wiser in ways I never expected. Not just about health. But about life. About choices. About consequences. About what really matters.

Before lupus, I thought I was invincible. I thought I could do anything. Eat anything. Stay up all night.

Party. Drink. Smoke. Fight. Whatever. And my body would just handle it. Bounce back. No problem. I was young. Strong. Healthy. Or so I thought.

But lupus shattered that illusion. Showed me: You're not invincible. You're human. Fragile. Mortal. And if you don't take care of yourself, your body will break down. And once it breaks down, it's hard to build back up.

Lupus taught me: Everything you put in your body matters. Food isn't just food. It's medicine. Or it's poison. Healthy food reduces inflammation. Heals. Strengthens. Junk food increases inflammation. Hurts. Weakens. Before lupus, I didn't care. Now? I read every label. I research every ingredient. I choose carefully. Because I know: one bad meal can trigger a week-long flare.

Stress kills. Literally. Before lupus, I'd let everything stress me out. Traffic. Arguments. Money. Work. People. Everything. And I thought it was normal. But lupus showed me: stress triggers flares. Stress weakens your immune system. Stress makes everything worse. So now, I manage stress. I avoid stressful situations. I remove stressful people. I practice breathing. Prayer. Meditation. Because my health depends on it.

Sleep is non-negotiable. Before lupus, I'd sleep four, five hours a night. Thought sleep was for the weak. But lupus taught me: your body heals when you sleep. Your immune system strengthens when you sleep. If you don't sleep, you don't heal. So now, I prioritize sleep.

Eight hours. Every night. No exceptions. And I feel the difference.

People affect your health. Toxic people create toxic stress. Drama. Negativity. Problems. And all of that affects your body. So I cut off toxic people. Set boundaries. Protect my peace. Because my health is more important than anyone's feelings.

Doctors aren't God. They don't have all the answers. They make mistakes. They misdiagnose. They prescribe wrong things. So I had to become my own advocate. Learn about lupus. Research treatments. Ask questions. Get second opinions. Because it's my body. My health. My responsibility.

Prevention is better than cure. It's easier to avoid a flare than to recover from one. So I do everything I can to prevent flares. Eat right. Sleep right. Manage stress. Take meds. Stay out of the sun. Stay out of extreme temperatures. It's not fun. But it works.

Life is short. And unpredictable. Lupus could have killed me. Could still kill me. So I don't waste time anymore. I don't hold grudges. I don't put off dreams. I don't wait for "someday." I live now. Love now. Create now. Because tomorrow isn't promised.

That's how lupus made me wiser. By showing me what I was too stubborn to see before. By forcing me to grow up. To take responsibility. To value life. To appreciate health. To make better choices. And I'm grateful for that. As painful as it's been, I'm grateful.

What's the biggest change in my character since being diagnosed with lupus?

My biggest change in my character is:

Once I see any signs of nonsense, I get away very fast. I waste no time around anyone who's talking nonsense. Doing nonsense.

I try my best to stop getting myself involved with someone who doesn't mean me well in life.

I don't deal with anyone who doesn't respect me or my business skills.

I try to keep an attitude of not dealing with anyone who can't help me like I help them while being in a position to be a sort of help.

The biggest change in my character? Zero tolerance for nonsense. That's it. That's the change. And it's saved my life.

Before lupus, I'd tolerate anything. Drama. Disrespect. Toxicity. People using me. People draining me. People wasting my time. I'd put up with it. Make excuses for them. Give them second chances. Third chances. A hundred chances. Because I didn't want to be mean. Didn't want to hurt feelings. Didn't want to lose friendships.

But lupus taught me: tolerating nonsense costs you your health. Your peace. Your energy. Your life. So I stopped.

Now: If someone is constantly negative, I remove them. No explanation. No argument. Just distance. Because negativity is contagious. And I can't afford to catch it.

If someone disrespects me, they're done. One chance. That's it. Disrespect me once, shame on you. Give you a second chance to do it again? Shame on me. So there are no second chances anymore.

If someone is always creating drama, I don't engage. I don't get involved. I don't take sides. I just step back. Let them figure it out. Because drama creates stress. And stress triggers flares. And flares put me in the hospital. So no drama. Period.

If someone only calls when they need something, I don't answer. I'm not a bank. I'm not a therapist. I'm not a rescue service. Friendship is mutual. If you only show up when you need help, you're not a friend. You're a user. And I don't have time for users.

If someone doesn't respect my business, my hustle, my grind, they can't be in my circle. I work hard. I'm building something. And if you can't support it, respect it, or at least not tear it down, then you can't be around me. Because I need people who lift me up. Not people who drag me down.

This might sound harsh. Cold. Mean. But it's not. It's self-preservation. It's survival. It's choosing life over being liked. Choosing health over being nice. Choosing peace over being popular.

And the people who really love me? They understand. They respect it. They adjust. Because they want me healthy. They want me alive. They want me thriving.

The people who don't understand? They're the ones I needed to remove anyway. So it all works out.

That's the biggest change. Zero tolerance for nonsense. And I'm not apologizing for it. Because it's keeping me alive.

Do I ever wonder what my life would be like if I'd never been diagnosed with lupus?

I think about it all the time. 24/7.

I think about the sports I'd be professional in. I think about the professional field of work.

I think about how stress-free, without a lot of ups and downs, my living situation would be.

I think about what state I'd be settling down in to grow old and happy.

I think about all the dreams I could have fulfilled in my life.

I think about how I would have been as a pro boxer. Every time I watch a boxing match on TV.

I think about how I could have had my own cooking show on TV or restaurant in my hometown.

So yes, I am always thinking about how my life would have been like and where I would have been in life.

Do I wonder? Every single day. Every single moment. Especially when I see what I could have been.

I watch boxing matches on TV. And I see fighters my age. Doing what I was supposed to do. Fighting professionally. Making money. Making a name. Living the dream. And I think: That could have been me. That should have been me. Pretty Boy the boxer. On TV. In the ring. Champion. If lupus hadn't taken it from me.

I see cooking shows. Chefs with their own restaurants. Their own shows. Their own brands. And I think: I could cook better than some of them. I have skills. I have creativity. I have passion. I could have had my own restaurant. Johnny's Kitchen. In Paterson. Packed every night. Lines out the door. If lupus hadn't changed my path.

I think about the money I'd be making. Professional boxer. Or celebrity chef. Or both. I'd be financially secure. No struggles. No stress. Nice house. Nice car. Traveling. Enjoying life. Providing for my family. If lupus hadn't limited me.

I think about my health. How I'd wake up without pain. Without stiffness. Without wondering if today would be a good day or a bad day. How I'd just live. Normal. Free. Unrestricted. How I'd play with my grandkids without worrying about getting too tired. How I'd work all day without needing to rest. How I'd just be. If lupus hadn't invaded my body.

I think about the dreams I had to let go. The career I had to abandon. The future I had to reimagine. And yeah, it hurts. It's loss. It's grief. It's mourning a life that could have been but never will be.

But here's what I also think:

Would I have changed without lupus? Probably not. I was on a bad path. Hanging with the wrong people. Making wrong choices. Heading toward prison. Or death. Or a wasted life. Lupus forced me to change. Forced me to choose better. Forced me to become who I am now.

Would I have found God without lupus? Maybe. Eventually. But probably not this deeply. Not this personally. Not with this level of faith and dependence. Lupus drove me to God. Made me need Him. Made me rely on Him. And that relationship? That's the most valuable thing I have.

Would I have appreciated life without lupus? No. I'd take it for granted. Waste it. Chase things that don't matter. But lupus taught me: life is precious. Health is a gift. Every good day is a blessing. And that perspective? That's priceless.

Would I be the person I am without lupus? No. Lupus shaped me. Made me wiser. Made me kinder. Made me more patient. More understanding. More grateful. More purposeful. And I like who I am now. I'm proud of who I am now. Even if I'm not who I thought I'd be.

So do I wonder what life would be like without lupus? Yes. All the time. But do I regret getting lupus? That's complicated. Because lupus took things from me. But it also gave me things. Things I wouldn't have gotten any other way. Wisdom. Faith. Character. Purpose. Perspective.

And maybe that's the answer. Maybe God didn't bless me with lupus to punish me. But to save me. To redirect me. To make me who I was supposed to be all along. Not a boxer. Not a chef. But a survivor. A testimony. A living example that you can lose everything and still find something. That you can be broken and still be beautiful. That you can have lupus and still have life. Abundant life. Meaningful life. Purposeful life.

That's what I think about when I wonder. Not just what could have been. But what is. And what will be. Because lupus changed my story. But it didn't end it. It just started a new chapter. And I'm still writing it. One day at a time.

So for the record, yes, I believe God put lupus in my life to make me a better person.

And it is one of the biggest reasons why I had to make lupus my guardian angel in some ways.

To always remind me from where I come from. When I discovered it will be part of my life for the rest of my life. And we will have to work together to survive this journey as long as we both can.

So did God bless me with lupus to make me a wiser person? Yes. Absolutely. Without a doubt.

Not because God wanted me to suffer. But because God wanted me to survive. To thrive. To become who He created me to be. And I was too stubborn to get there any other way.

Lupus is my guardian angel. That sounds crazy. How can a disease be a guardian angel? But it is. Because it guards me. It reminds me. It keeps me in check. It won't let me go back to who I was. It won't let me make the same mistakes. It won't let me take life for granted.

When I'm tempted to eat junk, lupus reminds me: That will hurt. Don't do it. When I'm tempted to skip meds, lupus reminds me: You need those. Take them. When I'm tempted to stress about things that don't matter, lupus reminds me: That's not worth your health. Let it go. When I'm tempted to hang with the wrong people, lupus reminds me: They're bad for you. Walk away.

Lupus keeps me humble. Keeps me grateful. Keeps me focused. Keeps me dependent on God. Keeps me living right. Keeps me choosing wisely. Keeps me remembering: I almost died. I almost wasted my life. But God gave me another chance. And I'm not going to waste it.

So yes, God blessed me with lupus. Not to punish me. But to save me. To make me wiser. To make me better. To make me who I am today. Someone who values life. Who appreciates health. Who follows God. Who makes good choices. Who helps others. Who has purpose. Who has meaning. Who has a testimony.

And my testimony is this: Lupus tried to destroy me. But God used it to develop me. Lupus tried to end me.

But God used it to elevate me. Lupus tried to define me. But God used it to refine me.

I am not Johnny with lupus. I am Johnny because of lupus. Because lupus made me who God intended me to be all along. And for that, I'm grateful. Even on the hard days. Even on the painful days. Even on the days I wish things were different. I'm grateful. Because I'm alive. I'm here. I'm wiser. I'm better. I'm blessed.

That's my lupus. That's my problem. That's my blessing. And I'm living it every single day.

Chapter 16
Turning My Pain Into A Purpose

When my lupus is upset with me and causes me to be in so much pain just because I didn't let it control my life, I take the pain and use it for meditating therapy.

I put my body into a tight squeeze position and put my hands on the top of my chin and close my eyes and began praying so hard:

"Please let this pain pass through and keep it moving. Please. I refuse to let it take over my time and life for the future I am struggling to fight for."

I also say: "Come on, lupus. Please don't turn against me now. We have been through this for thirty years. Please, let's work together because you know by now I'm not giving up and letting you run things here. So please, let's get it together. We have a purpose. We still have goals we are trying to accomplish and achieve. There are people involved in our lives that need us. Like my fiancée and my daughter and grandkids and the new lives we are trying to bring in the world."

And so the lupus will start to ease up the pain and send it away for the time being.

And yes, I start to get up and get back on the mission and my journey.

This is how I deal with pain. Not with just medication. Not with just doctors. But with conversation. With negotiation. With partnership. Because lupus and I? We're in this together. Whether we like it or not. And I've learned: I can't fight lupus. I have to work with it. Talk to it. Reason with it. Make it understand: We're on the same side. We both want to survive. We both want to live. So let's stop fighting each other. And start fighting for each other.

That's my relationship with lupus. It's not an enemy. It's not a curse. It's my problem. My partner. My teacher. My reminder. And when the pain comes, when it gets unbearable, when it feels like lupus is punishing me, I don't get angry. I don't give up. I talk to it. I reason with it. I remind it: We've been through worse. We've survived thirty years. We're not stopping now. We have too much to live for. Too many people counting on us. Too many dreams to chase. Too much purpose to fulfill.

And most of the time? Lupus listens. The pain eases. The body calms. And I get back up. Back to the mission. Back to the journey. Back to living.

Can I describe my tight squeeze position when I am doing meditation techniques? And how I discovered it?

When I am meditating on something better for myself, I lay back in my bed with my arms crossed, my hands in the back of my head, with my legs crossed over each other, while wiggling my toes up and down.

And the longest I held this position is for about an hour.

And then I turn to another position. Like I will turn on my side and put one hand behind my head and one hand between my legs and scrunch up really tight because I would be in that much pain.

My pain would be over a ten.

And I would stay in that position for an hour or more.

Let me explain this meditation technique in more detail. Because it's not something I read in a book. It's not something a doctor taught me. It's something I discovered. Through trial and error. Through years of pain. Through desperate attempts to find relief when nothing else worked.

This is where I start. Lying flat on my back in bed. Arms crossed. Hands behind my head. Like I'm relaxing. But I'm not relaxing. I'm fighting. Fighting pain. Fighting inflammation. Fighting lupus.

My legs are crossed over each other. Right leg over left. Or left over right. Depends on which side hurts more. The crossing creates pressure. Compression. And somehow, that compression helps. It distracts from the deeper pain. Gives my mind something else to focus on.

And my toes? I wiggle them. Up and down. Up and down. Constantly. Why? I don't know. But it works.

The movement keeps me present. Keeps me focused. Keeps me from drowning in the pain. It's like a metronome. A rhythm. A beat that says: You're still here. You're still fighting. You're still alive.

I stay in this position for about an hour. Sometimes more. Sometimes less. Depends on the pain. Depends on how bad the flare is. Depends on whether lupus is listening to my conversation or ignoring me.

And while I'm in this position, I meditate. I pray. I talk to God. I talk to lupus. I visualize the pain leaving. I see it like a dark cloud. Heavy. Thick. Suffocating. And I breathe it out. Slowly. Deliberately. With each breath, the cloud gets lighter. Smaller. Less powerful. Until it's gone. Or at least manageable.

When the back position stops working, I switch. I turn onto my side. Usually my left side. Because my right side has more pain.

One hand goes behind my head. Supporting it. Keeping my neck aligned. The other hand goes between my legs. Pressed tight. Creating that same compression. That same distraction. That same relief.

And I scrunch up. Really tight. Fetal position. But tighter. More compressed. More contained. Like I'm trying to make myself as small as possible. Like I'm trying to protect myself from the pain. Or maybe trap the pain inside so it can't spread. I don't know. But it helps.

My pain at this point? It's beyond a ten. It's a ten plus. Maybe a fifteen. Maybe a twenty. Numbers don't matter anymore. It's just pain. Overwhelming. All-consuming. Unbearable. The kind of pain that makes you want to scream. Or cry. Or give up. But I don't. I scrunch up. I pray. I talk to lupus. And I wait. For the pain to ease. For the conversation to work. For relief to come.

I stay in this position for an hour. Sometimes more. Sometimes I fall asleep like this. And wake up hours later, still in the same position. Body stiff. Muscles cramped. But pain? A little less. A little more bearable. Enough to get up. Enough to keep going.

I didn't plan this. I didn't research this. I didn't learn this from anyone. It just happened. Out of desperation. Out of necessity. Out of years of trying everything else and nothing working.

In the early years of lupus, when the pain was new and terrifying, I'd try everything. Pain meds. Heat pads. Ice packs. Hot baths. Cold compresses. Lying still. Moving around. Nothing worked. Or if it worked, it didn't work for long. The pain always came back. Stronger. Meaner. More persistent.

And one night, during a really bad flare, I was lying in bed. In so much pain I couldn't move. Couldn't think. Couldn't do anything but hurt. And I just instinctively crossed my arms behind my head. Crossed my legs. Started wiggling my toes. And I don't know why. But it felt right. It felt like it was helping. So I stayed like that.

And I prayed. And I talked to lupus. And slowly, grad-ually, the pain eased. Not completely. But enough.

And from that night on, that became my technique. My position. My meditation. My conversation with lupus. It's not scientific. It's not proven. It's not in any medical textbook. But it's mine. And it works. For me. And that's all that matters.

Can I describe a time when my pain was really, really painful? It was when both my legs had open sores. I had rashes everywhere on my arms and face. My legs and toes were swollen up really big. And the pain was higher than any number I can think of. Instead of 10/10, it was a 20/20.

I would stay coiled up in my side position all day. Would go to sleep and wake up in the same position.

Let me explain what a 10/10 pain feels like. Because if you've never experienced it, you can't imagine it. You think you know pain. You've stubbed your toe. You've had a headache. You've pulled a muscle. But that's not 10/10 pain. That's not even close.

10/10 pain is when every nerve in your body is on fire. When every joint feels like it's being crushed. When every muscle feels like it's being ripped apart. When breathing hurts. When blinking hurts. When existing hurts. That's 10/10.

But what I experienced on my worst day? That wasn't 10/10. That was beyond. That was 20/20. If ten is the highest pain a human should be able to endure, I was double that. I was past endurance. Past tolerance. Past survival mode. I was in a place where pain becomes the only reality. Where nothing else exists. Where you can't think about anything else. Can't focus on anything else. Can't feel anything else. Just pain.

Here's what my body looked like on that day:

Both my legs had open sores. Not small sores. Not little cuts. But open, weeping wounds. From the varicose veins bursting. From the skin breaking down. From lupus attacking my circulatory system. The sores were raw. Painful. Infected. Every time I moved, they'd tear a little more. Bleed a little more. Hurt a little more.

I had rashes everywhere. On my arms. On my face. The butterfly rash across my nose and cheeks, bright red. Angry. Inflamed. Like my face was on fire. And my arms? Covered. Red patches. Raised bumps. Itchy. Burning. Both at the same time. It was torture.

My legs and toes were swollen up really big. My ankles were twice their normal size. My feet were so swollen I couldn't wear shoes. My toes looked like sausages. Thick. Tight. Shiny. The skin stretched so thin I thought it would split. And every time my heart beat, I could feel the blood pulsing in my swollen legs. Throbbing. Pounding. Adding to the pain.

And the pain? It wasn't just in one place. It was everywhere. Every joint. Every muscle. Every inch of skin. My whole body was one giant nerve ending screaming in agony. I couldn't move without crying out. Couldn't shift positions without wanting to die. Couldn't do anything but lie there and hurt.

So I stayed coiled up in my side position. All day. Didn't eat. Didn't drink. Didn't use the bathroom. Just stayed in that position. Praying. Talking to lupus. Begging God for relief. For mercy. For the pain to stop. For death, if that's what it took. Because living with that pain didn't feel like living. It felt like dying. Slowly. Painfully. Endlessly.

I went to sleep like that. Or maybe I passed out. I don't know. But when I woke up, I was in the same position. Body stiff. Muscles cramped. But still coiled up. Still protecting myself. Still surviving.

That was my 20/20 day. And I pray I never have another one like it. But if I do, I know what to do. Coil up. Pray. Talk to lupus. And survive. Because that's all I can do. Survive.

How often do I have these conversations with lupus?

Very often.

To let it know: "I know you're still in my life. But I am still in control. Yes, you're my lupus but my problem."

I talk to lupus every single day. Not always out loud. But in my head. In my heart. In my spirit. It's a constant conversation. A constant negotiation. A constant reminder: We're in this together. But I'm in charge.

Every morning when I wake up, I check in. "How are we doing today, lupus? You going to cooperate? Or are you going to make this difficult?" And I listen. I feel. I assess. If my joints are stiff, I know lupus is awake and active. If my skin is itchy, I know inflammation is building. If I feel that deep fatigue, I know a flare might be coming. And I adjust. I plan. I prepare.

Throughout the day, I talk to it. When I'm tempted to eat something I shouldn't, I remind lupus: "You know that's going to hurt us both. Let's make a better choice." When I'm tempted to skip my meds, I reason with it: "These meds are keeping us alive. Let's take them." When I'm stressed, I acknowledge it: "I know this is hard. I know you don't like stress. Let me calm down. Let me breathe. Let's get through this together."

At night, before bed, I recap. "We made it through another day, lupus. Good job. Thank you for easing up when I needed it. Thank you for letting me function. Let's rest now. Let's heal. And tomorrow, we'll do it again."

And when the pain comes? When the flares hit? When lupus gets angry? I don't get angry back. I don't curse it. I don't hate it. I talk to it. I reason with it. Like I'm talking to a scared child. Or a stubborn friend. Or a partner who's having a bad day.

"Come on, lupus. Please don't turn against me now. We have been through this for thirty years. Please, let's work together because you know by now I'm not giving up and letting you run things here. So please, let's get it together. We have a purpose. We still have goals we are trying to accomplish and achieve. There are people that are involved in our lives that need us. Like my fiancée and my daughter and grandkids and the new lives we are trying to bring in the world."

And most of the time, lupus listens. The pain eases. The inflammation calms. The flare passes. Not because of the meds. Not because of the position. But because of the conversation. Because I acknowledged it. Respected it. Reminded it: We're on the same team. Let's act like it.

That's how often I have these conversations. Every day. Multiple times a day. It's not weird. It's not crazy. It's survival. It's partnership. It's the only way I know how to live with this disease. By talking to it. By working with it. By making it my problem. Not my enemy. My problem. And problems? You can solve problems. You can manage problems. You can live with problems. As long as you're willing to work together.

I also have my daughter Shakia Thomas and grandkids Naveah and Nyla Thomas.

My daughter is very independent, thank God for that, because what I am dealing with living with lupus is enough to take care of on its own.

My grandkids are both deeply involved in church with their grandmother and their cousins. They always perform praise dances in many different churches, and Nyla also sings solo in many different states.

My oldest granddaughter Naveah loves to dance and play drums and study digital creations. My youngest granddaughter Nyla loves to dance and sing and is really good. She has done many different church gospel concerts and holiday plays.

Let me tell you more about these four most important people in my life. Because they're not just family. They're my reason. My purpose. My why. When the pain gets unbearable, when lupus gets too strong, when I want to give up, I think about them. And I keep going.

My true love, my fiancée, she is everything I hoped she'd be. My daughter Shakia Thomas is strong. Independent. Confident. She doesn't need me to survive. She's built her own life, has her own lifestyle going on, her own path. I am proud of her that she can stand on her own.

She loves to hang out on weekends. Go to clubs. Go to concerts. She enjoys her life. And she loves her rap music. The kind I don't understand. The kind that's too fast, too loud, too much for my taste. But she loves it. And when she's in the car with me, that's what we listen to. Her music. And I don't complain. Because seeing her happy? That's worth any music I don't like.

And when a special day or holiday comes around, we all try to get together. Me, my daughter, my fiancée and grandkids. We try to do a dinner and movie and catch up with what's going on with everyone. To see if everyone is okay and doing what they're supposed to do in life. To make sure they're alright.

And when I can, I try to do one on one time with my grandkids also. Like with my oldest granddaughter Naveah Thomas. I make sure she's on the right track and doing what she's supposed to do to keep good grades in school. And I always ask her what she plans to be when she grows up.

She studies digital creations. Graphic design. Video editing. Animation. She's always on the computer. Creating. Building. Designing. And I don't understand half of what she's doing. But I support it. As long as it's positive.

And you know what she tells me? "Grandpa, when I grow up, I'm going to make a video about you. About your life. About lupus. About how you never gave up." And I believe her. Because that's who she is. Thoughtful. Creative. Loving. And if she does make that video? I'll be the proudest grandpa in the world.

And my youngest granddaughter Nyla Thomas. She's a star. Not just in my eyes but in everyone's eyes. She loves to dance. Loves to sing. And she's really good. Not "good for a little girl." Just good. Period. Her voice is clear. Strong. Confident. She doesn't get nervous. Doesn't get shy. She gets on stage and she performs. Like she was born to do it.

She's done many different church gospel concerts. Holiday plays. Christmas programs. Easter services. Wherever there's a stage and a microphone, Nyla's there. Singing. Dancing. Praising God. And the church loves her. The community loves her. I love her.

Both my grandkids love gospel music. Love going to church. Not because I force them. Not because their parents make them. But because they genuinely love it. They feel God. They worship. They praise. And seeing them so young, so committed, so full of faith? It gives me hope. Hope that they'll never lose that. Hope that God will protect them. Guide them. Bless them. The way He's protected, guided, and blessed me.

They all like me to cook their favorite food. When they come over to my house, the first thing they ask: "Grandpa, what you cooking?" And I make them whatever they want. Whatever. Because cooking for them? That's love. That's legacy. That's me passing down something. Not just recipes. But tradition. Culture. Care. The knowledge that food is more than food. It's connection. It's family. It's love on a plate.

These four are my world. My reason for fighting. My reason for talking to lupus. My reason for getting up every day. Even when the pain says stay down. Even when the body says quit. Even when lupus says it's over. I think about them. And I keep going. Because they need me. And I need them. And that's enough. More than enough. That's everything.

So you ask me what new lives I am trying to bring in the world. I am praying for a son and another daughter if God puts it in His will.

I know I have lupus. I'm not supposed to be thinking about more kids. But I am. Because life isn't over. Because my purpose isn't fulfilled. Because I still have love to give. Still have lessons to teach. Still have legacy to build.

My fiancée and I talk about it. About having a child together. A son. A daughter. Maybe both. And people look at us like we're crazy. "You're too old. You're too sick. You can't handle more kids." But they don't understand. This isn't about what I can handle. This is about what I want. What I dream. What I pray for.

I want a big family. Because I always wanted that more than anything. To show different paths. To pass down different lessons. I want to teach them how to be independent. Who provides for their family. Who stands up for their rights. Who doesn't give up when life gets hard. Who fights through pain. Who turns problems into purpose.

I want a big family because the world needs more good, strong, positive men and women.

Is it realistic? I don't know. Is it medically advisable? Probably not. Is it possible? Only God knows. But I'm praying for it. I'm believing for it. I'm preparing for it. Because if God puts it in His will, if God opens that door, if God blesses me with more children, I'm ready. Lupus and all. Pain and all. Age and all. I'm ready. Because being a father? That's the best thing I've ever done. And if I get to do it again? That would be the greatest blessing. The greatest purpose. The greatest legacy.

What did I do when lupus didn't ease up at some times? I work out. I did my stretching routine. I did my exercise bike. I punched my punching bag. I've done all these things. And after a while, it did ease up.

Let me clarify something. Sometimes, the conversation doesn't work. Sometimes, the tight squeeze position doesn't help. Sometimes, lupus doesn't listen. And when that happens, I don't just lie there. I fight. Differently. More aggressively. More physically.

I work out. Not the way I used to. Not 750 pullups. Not three-hour runs. But enough. Enough to move the blood. Enough to loosen the joints. Enough to remind my body: We're still capable. We're still strong. We're still fighters.

My stretching routine: I start slow. Gentle. I stretch my neck. Side to side. Up and down. Then my shoulders. Rolling them. Loosening them. Then my back. Twisting. Bending. Then my legs. Hamstrings. Quads. Calves. Every muscle. Every joint. Slowly. Carefully. Because if I push too hard, I'll make it worse. But if I don't move at all, the stiffness will win. So I stretch. For twenty minutes. Thirty minutes. Sometimes an hour. Until something gives. Until something loosens. Until the pain eases just a little.

My exercise bike: This is my cardio. My low-impact movement. I can't run anymore. Can't jump. Can't do high-impact exercise. But I can bike. Slowly. Steadily. I set the resistance low. Pedal at a comfortable pace. And I go. For fifteen minutes. Twenty minutes. Sometimes thirty. And as I pedal, I feel it. The blood moving. The joints loosening. The inflammation decreasing. Not completely. But enough. Enough to remind me: Movement is medicine. Activity is healing. Even with lupus. Even with pain. Keep moving. And you keep living.

My punching bag: This is my therapy. My release. My fight. I can't box anymore. Can't spar. Can't compete. But I can still hit. And when lupus is being stubborn, when the pain won't leave, when I'm frustrated and angry and tired of dealing with this disease, I hit the bag. Not hard. Not like I used to. But enough. Enough to feel powerful. Enough to feel strong. Enough to release the anger. The frustration. The fear. Jab. Jab. Right hand. Left hook. Body shot. Over and over. Until I'm tired. Until I'm sweating. Until the endorphins kick in. And the pain? It's still there. But it's less. Because I fought back. Because I didn't just surrender. Because I reminded lupus: I'm still Pretty Boy. I'm still a fighter. And you're not going to beat me.

Yes, I've done all these things. And after a while, the pain did ease up. Not always. Not every time. But often enough. Often enough to know: when the conversation doesn't work, when the position doesn't help, when nothing else is working, I have options. I have tools. I have ways to fight back. And I will use them. Every single one. Because giving up isn't an option. Surrendering isn't an option. I'm going to fight. Every day. Every way I know how. Until lupus eases up. Or until I can't fight anymore. Whichever comes first.

What gives me the strength when nothing else is working for me?

My fiancée. My daughter. My grandkids.

Thinking about what will happen to them if I'm not around. How will they feel.

I think about all their smiles when spending time with them.

I think about all the things we plan to do that we didn't get to do yet.

I think about all the exciting things I want to do with them also. And that's what keeps me going and gives me my strength.

When nothing else works, when the pain won't stop, when the conversation fails, when the position doesn't help, when the workout doesn't ease it, when I've tried everything and nothing is working, I think about them. My family. My reason. My purpose. And somehow, that's enough. That gives me strength. Not physical strength. But something deeper. Spiritual strength. The strength to endure. To survive. To keep going even when everything in me wants to stop.

I think about my fiancée. About what would happen if I wasn't here. Who would she lean on? Who would she talk to? Who would make her laugh when she's stressed? Who would cook for her? Who would pray with her? Who would remind her she's beautiful when she doesn't feel beautiful? Me. That's who. So I have to stay. I have to keep fighting. I have to survive. Because she needs me. And I need her. And that need? That's stronger than pain. That's stronger than lupus. That's stronger than anything this disease can throw at me.

I think about my daughter. About what would happen if I died. How would she feel? Would she blame herself? Would she think she didn't do enough? Would she be okay? Would she be strong? I raised her to be strong. But losing a parent? That's different. That changes you. And I don't want her to have to go through that yet. Not yet. I want more time. More Sunday dinners. More conversations. More hugs. More "I love you, Dad." More years. So I keep fighting. Because she's not ready to lose me. And I'm not ready to leave her.

I think about my grandkids. About all their smiles when spending time with them. When I pick them up. When I cook for them. When I watch them perform. When I tell them I'm proud. When I pray with them. Those smiles? They are everything. They are what life is about. Not money. Not success. Not fame. But those smiles. That joy. That love. That connection. And if I give up, if I stop fighting, if I let lupus win, I don't get to see those smiles anymore. I don't get to hear them call me Grandpa. I don't get to watch them grow. I don't get to be part of their story. And that's unacceptable. So I fight. For those smiles. For those moments. For them.

I think about all the things we plan to do that we didn't get to do yet. Vacations we haven't taken. Holidays we haven't celebrated. Birthdays we haven't reached. Milestones we haven't witnessed. Naveah graduating high school. Nyla's first recital. Shakia's wedding. Future grandkids. Great-grandkids. All of it. All the things I want to experience. All the moments I want to share. All the memories I want to make. We planned them. We talked about them. We dreamed about them. And I'll be damned if lupus takes those away. So I keep fighting. Because those plans are still on the table. Those dreams are still alive. And as long as I'm alive, they're possible.

I think about all the exciting things I want to do with them also. Teaching Naveah to cook. Teaching Nyla about music. Teaching my future son about boxing. Teaching my future daughter about strength. Showing them all what it means to never give up. What it means to fight through pain. What it means to turn your problem into your purpose. Those are the things I want to do. Those are the lessons I want to pass down. That's the legacy I want to leave. And I can't do any of that if I'm gone. So I stay. I fight. I survive. For them. For me. For all of us.

That's what keeps me going. That's what gives me my strength. When nothing else works, when I've tried everything, when I'm at my lowest, when I want to give up, I think about them. And I find the strength to keep going. One more day. One more hour. One more minute. Whatever it takes. Because they're worth it. Because life is worth it. Because this fight is worth it. And I'll keep fighting until I can't fight anymore. And even then, I'll probably try to fight a little more. Because that's what fighters do. That's what fathers do. That's what grandpas do. That's what I do.

I believe when a person is not listening to his parents at a time in life, or not doing the right thing at some point in time, I believe God will let you see what is possible for you in the nearest future. And that is health issues and pain.

I've felt like pain had a purpose. Many times. Almost every day. Because if pain doesn't have a purpose, then it's just suffering. And I can't accept that. I can't accept that I'm going through all of this for nothing. There has to be a reason. There has to be meaning. There has to be purpose.

And I believe the purpose is this: God was trying to get my attention. God was trying to wake me up. God was trying to redirect me. Before it was too late. Before I ended up dead. Or in prison. Or wasting my entire life.

When I was young, I wasn't listening. To my mom. To my elders. To God. I was hanging with the wrong people. Making wrong choices. Doing wrong things. And I thought I was untouchable. I thought I could get away with it forever. But God had other plans. God said: "If you won't listen to your mom, if you won't listen to your conscience, if you won't listen to Me through words, then I'll speak through pain. Through health issues. Through consequences you can't ignore."

And that's what happened. At twenty-six, my body started breaking down. Symptoms appeared. Pain started. Lupus was diagnosed. And suddenly, I couldn't ignore it anymore. I had to pay attention. I had to listen. I had to change. Because if I didn't, I would die. Simple as that.

So the purpose of the pain? It was intervention. It was correction. It was redirection. God using lupus to save my life. To force me to stop. To make me think. To give me a choice: Continue down this path and die. Or change and live.

And I chose to live. I chose to change. I chose to listen. And yes, the pain is still here. The lupus is still here. But so am I. Still alive. Still fighting. Still growing. Still learning. Still becoming who God intended me to be. And that wouldn't have happened without the pain. Without lupus. Without this disease forcing me to confront myself. Forcing me to choose better. Forcing me to find purpose.

So yes, pain has a purpose. It's not random. It's not meaningless. It's not just suffering. It's God's megaphone. God's wake-up call. God's intervention. And I'm grateful for it. Even though it hurts. Even though it's hard. Even though I wish things were different. I'm grateful. Because the pain saved my life. And now, I'm using the pain to fulfill my purpose. To help others. To inspire others. To show others: You can have pain and still have purpose. You can have lupus and still have life. You can suffer and still have meaning. That's the purpose. That's why I'm still here. That's why I keep fighting. To turn my pain into purpose. And to help others do the same.

I want my legacy to be that no matter what position you are in with health issues; mentally, physically or financially, still be happy for living life and keep trying for better.

In your life, don't give up on yourself or God.

And I want all my kids and anyone who was for me in my life to be and feel the same.

I just want to leave behind a good legacy no matter what.

My legacy. That's what this is all about, isn't it? Not the pain. Not the lupus. Not the struggle. But what I leave behind when I'm gone. What people remember. What lessons they carry. What impact I made. That's legacy. And I think about it a lot. More than I probably should. But when you have a disease that could kill you at any time, you think about legacy. You think about what you're leaving. You think about whether your life mattered.

And here's what I want my legacy to be:

I want people to say: "Johnny never gave up. No matter how hard it got. No matter how much pain he was in. No matter how many times lupus knocked him down. He got back up. Every single time. He kept fighting. He kept believing. He kept going. And that inspired me. That showed me I can keep going too."

I want my kids and grandkids to say: "Grandpa taught us that life isn't about what happens to you. It's about what you do with what happens. He had lupus. He had pain. He had struggles. But he didn't let that define him. He defined himself. He chose joy. He chose purpose. He chose to keep trying. And we learned that from him. We carry that with us. That's his gift to us."

I want people with chronic illness to say: "Johnny showed me it's possible. To have a disease and still have a life. To be in pain and still have purpose. To struggle and still be happy. He proved it's not about the circumstances. It's about the attitude. It's about the fight. It's about refusing to let your problem become your prison. He turned his problem into his purpose. And if he can do it, maybe I can too."

I want people who knew me before lupus to say: "Johnny changed. He was heading down a bad path. But something happened. Something woke him up. Something made him turn around. And he became a better man. A wiser man. A stronger man. Not despite lupus. But because of it. He let God use the pain to transform him. And that transformation was beautiful."

I want my legacy to be that no matter what position you are in with health issues; mentally, physically or financially, still be happy for living life and keep trying for better. Don't give up. Don't quit. Don't let your circumstances define you. You define your circumstances. You decide what they mean. You decide what you do with them. You decide whether they destroy you or develop you. That's the choice. That's the power. That's the legacy.

In your life, don't give up on yourself or God. Because when you give up on yourself, you lose hope. And when you give up on God, you lose faith. And without hope and faith, life becomes unbearable. But with hope and faith? With the belief that things can get better? With the trust that God has a plan? With the conviction that your life has purpose? Then you can endure anything. You can survive anything. You can overcome anything. That's what I want people to know. That's what I want people to remember. That's my legacy.

And I want all my kids and anyone who was for me in my life to be and feel the same. To carry that mindset. To live that truth. To pass it down. To their kids. To their friends. To anyone who's struggling. To keep the legacy alive. Not just as my story. But as their story. Our story. The story of people who refused to give up. Who turned pain into purpose. Who found meaning in suffering. Who lived with joy despite circumstances. That's the legacy. That's what I'm building. That's what I'm fighting for. Every single day.

I just want to leave behind a good legacy no matter what. Not perfect. Not flawless. Not without mistakes. But good. Honest. Real. A legacy that says: He lived. He struggled. He suffered. But he kept going. He kept believing. He kept fighting. And in the end, his life mattered. Not because he was famous. Not because he was rich. Not because he was successful by the world's standards. But because he loved well. He fought hard. He never gave up. And he showed others how to do the same. That's a good legacy. That's the legacy I want. And with God's help, with lupus as my teacher, with pain as my purpose, that's the legacy I'll leave. No matter what.

Chapter 17
The Shocking News of My Community

Well, like I was saying in the beginning and towards the middle of this story on my life, how it took me so many different doctors and my own personal natural remedies to figure out how can I get this lupus under control and stable enough to want to deal with.

At the same time, how can I keep up my faith into wanting to even go on in life.

And after I figured out how to control my lupus, I started to feel like this lifestyle is my new normal. Watching out on everything I do with myself in life, from physical to mental.

How long did I hide my lupus? And for how long?

Well, I didn't hide it like I didn't want anyone to know. It was people who started asking me how I hide lupus because I was maintaining it so well. They were just surprised once I started telling people I have it.

The people I told knew all about lupus before I told them because of a family member of theirs. So this is the reason they started saying if I would have never said I had lupus, they would never be able to tell I had it.

Let me be clear about something: I didn't hide lupus intentionally. I wasn't trying to keep it a secret. I wasn't ashamed. I wasn't embarrassed. I just wasn't advertising it. There's a difference.

When you first get diagnosed with a chronic illness, you don't know how to talk about it. You don't know who to tell. You don't know when to tell. You don't know how people will react. So you keep it to yourself. Not because you're hiding. But because you're processing. You're learning. You're adjusting. You're figuring out your new normal before you invite others into it.

And that's what I did. For the first few years after diagnosis, I kept lupus to myself. I told my immediate family. My mom. My siblings. The people who needed to know. But friends? Coworkers? Acquaintances? I didn't tell them. Not yet. Not until I understood what I was dealing with. Not until I learned how to manage it. Not until I felt confident enough to explain it.

And by the time I started telling people, I had figured it out. I had learned how to control it. How to manage the symptoms. How to prevent flares. How to live a relatively normal life despite having lupus. So when I finally started opening up, people were shocked. Not because I had lupus. But because I had been managing it so well they couldn't tell.

They said things like: "If you never told me, I would have never known." "You don't look sick." "How are you keeping yourself up like that without showing any signs?"

And I realized: I wasn't hiding lupus. I was maintaining it. There's a difference. Hiding means keeping it secret out of shame or fear. Maintaining means managing it so well that it doesn't define you. And that's what I did. I maintained lupus. I kept it under control. I didn't let it take over my life. And because of that, people couldn't tell. Not because I was hiding it. But because I was winning against it.

And as time went on in my journey, some of the individuals who I were friends with, to who I was in a relationship with, to who I had business with, they never knew or had any idea what I was dealing with.

The first time I told a person I have lupus was my fiancée when we had a year into the relationship.

When I first told her, she didn't have any knowledge on lupus either. So she ended up doing research on lupus so she could learn about it and be of help towards me with dealing with lupus.

It made me very, very, very happy and proud. I knew that God had to put her in my life. Because that is probably anyone's fear: dealing with a disease that can't be cured and is just treatable. It's hard to find someone who wants to be in a long-term relationship or just being involved with someone's living situation while trying to help them manage their health issues.

So me and my fiancée both just took it on ourselves to search for the best rheumatologist and natural treatment substances to help me manage my lupus.

Let me tell you about that conversation. Because it was one of the most important conversations of my life.

We had been together for a year. A whole year. And she didn't know. Not because I was hiding it. But because I was scared. Scared she'd leave. Scared she'd see me differently. Scared she'd think I was damaged goods. Scared she wouldn't want to deal with a man who has a chronic illness. Who might have bad days. Who might need help. Who might not be able to do all the things a "normal" man can do.

But after a year, I knew I had to tell her. Because you can't build a real relationship on secrets. You can't build trust on half-truths. You can't build a future with someone who doesn't know the whole you. So I decided: I'm going to tell her. And whatever happens, happens. If she leaves, she leaves. If she stays, she stays. But she deserves to know.

We were sitting in my living room. Just talking. Watching TV. Normal evening. And I turned the TV off. And she looked at me like, "What's wrong?" And I said, "I need to tell you something. Something important. Something I should have told you a long time ago."

And I could see the worry on her face. Like she thought I was about to break up with her. Or tell her I cheated. Or some other relationship-ending news.

And I said: "I have lupus. I was diagnosed years ago. And I've been managing it. But I should have told you sooner. And I'm sorry I didn't. But I'm telling you now. Because you deserve to know. And if this is too much for you, if you don't want to deal with this, I understand. I won't be mad. I won't hold it against you. But I need you to know what you're getting into if you stay with me."

And she just looked at me. For what felt like forever. Not saying anything. Just looking. And I thought: This is it. She's going to leave. She's going to say it's too much. She's going to walk away. And I braced myself for it.

But then she said: "What's lupus?"

And I almost laughed. Not because it was funny. But because I was expecting rejection. And instead, I got curiosity. She didn't know what lupus was. She had never heard of it. So she wasn't scared of it. She wasn't making assumptions. She just wanted to know.

So I explained it. As best I could. It's an autoimmune disease. My immune system attacks my own body. It causes inflammation. Pain. Fatigue. Rashes. Organ damage if not managed. There's no cure. But it's treatable. With medication. With lifestyle changes. With careful management. And I've been doing that successfully for years. That's why she couldn't tell. That's why I seemed normal. Because I worked hard to maintain it.

And she listened. Asked questions. Good questions. "Is it contagious?" No. "Did you get it from someone?" Kind of. It's genetic. "Can you die from it?" Yes. If not managed. But I'm managing it. "What do you need from me?" Just understanding. Patience. Support when I'm having bad days. That's it.

And then she said: "Okay. I'm going to learn about this. I'm going to research it. So I can understand what you're dealing with. And I'm going to help you. However I can. Because I love you. And this doesn't change that. You're still you. Lupus is just something you have. It's not who you are."

And I cried. Right there. In front of her. Because that's the response I needed. That's the acceptance I was hoping for. That's the support I was scared I wouldn't get. And she gave it. Without hesitation. Without judgment. Without fear. Just love. Just commitment. Just partnership.

And she kept her word. She researched lupus. Read articles. Watched videos. Joined support groups. Learned about symptoms. About triggers. About treatments. And then she helped me. Helped me find better doctors. Better rheumatologists. Better natural treatments. She became my partner in managing lupus. Not just my girlfriend. But my partner. My teammate. My support system.

And that's when I knew: God put her in my life for a reason. Because finding someone who will stay when things get hard? Who will learn about your disease? Who will help you manage it? Who will love you despite it? That's rare. That's a blessing. That's everything.

What physical signs or symptoms do people notice about me?

Well, I think the first symptoms will appear in my face around my eyes. Because the first thing they will say is: "Are you feeling okay?"

I ask, "Why?"

They say: "Because you don't look too healthy in the face. Your eyes are really reddish. Your face is really reddish and very, very dry and flaky."

The face always gives it away. That's the first thing people notice. When lupus is active, when I'm having a flare, when things are getting bad, my face shows it. Even when I'm trying to hide it. Even when I'm putting on a brave face. My actual face betrays me.

My eyes get red. Not just a little bloodshot. But really red. Inflamed. Like I've been crying. Or like I haven't slept in days. Or like I'm sick. People notice. They ask: "Are you okay? Your eyes look bad. Are you getting enough sleep? Are you sick? Do you have allergies?" And I have to decide: Do I tell them? Do I explain? Or do I brush it off?

My face gets red too. The butterfly rash. That's the classic lupus symptom. Redness across the nose and cheeks in the shape of a butterfly. Sometimes it's subtle. Just a little pink. Sometimes it's obvious. Bright red. Angry. Inflamed. Like I got sunburned. But I wasn't in the sun. It's just lupus. Attacking my skin. Making itself known.

And my face gets very, very dry and flaky. The skin peels. Cracks. Bleeds sometimes. No amount of lotion helps. No amount of moisturizer makes a difference. It's not regular dry skin. It's lupus dry skin. It's inflammation. It's the disease attacking my skin cells. And it shows. People notice. They comment. They suggest products. "Have you tried this lotion? Have you tried drinking more water? Have you tried a humidifier?" And I appreciate it. But it's not that simple. It's lupus. And lupus doesn't care about lotion.

So yes, the face is the first giveaway. When people say: "Are you feeling okay?" They're seeing what I'm feeling. They're noticing what I'm trying to hide. And that's when I have to decide: Do I open up? Do I explain? Do I tell them about lupus? Or do I just say: "I'm fine. Just tired." And keep moving.

When I got a little weird at some times, didn't want to talk much, not so hyped when I heard someone else's success, all the way until I shut down and shied away from people, didn't answer my phone, my texts, didn't just want to be bothered until I started feeling myself getting back strong or feeling healthy.

How do I explain lupus to someone who doesn't have it?

Well, usually when I am telling someone I have lupus and they seem confused and shocked, and sometimes they think it's a catchy disease.

So I explain to them it is an immune disorder. And you do not catch it from someone. You inherit it from someone in your family. It can come from your mother's side or father's side of the family. And sometimes it can skip siblings and be inherited to the youngest of the family member.

You can still live a healthy lifestyle as long as your track record stays fresh and updated with your family of doctors and specialists. And I mean like everything that the lupus can affect on the body and organs.

Like first, you will get yourself a primary doctor for regular routine checkups. You will get yourself a dermatologist so they can keep your skin looking healthy. Then you will get yourself a nutritionist for a healthy diet. A kidney specialist to keep watch on your kidneys. You will get yourself a dentist to keep up with your teeth. And most of all, your almighty rheumatologist, the king or queen of keeping the lupus stable enough to want to deal with trying to do better with your health.

That is your very own family of doctors.

Explaining lupus to someone who's never heard of it is hard. Because it's complicated. It's not like a cold. Or the flu. Or cancer. It's different. It's invisible. It's unpredictable. It's confusing. Even for the person who has it. So explaining it to someone who doesn't? That's a challenge.

Here's how I explain it:

"Lupus is an autoimmune disease. That means my immune system, which is supposed to protect me from sickness, attacks me instead. It attacks my own body. My own organs. My own tissues. It doesn't know the difference between a virus and my own cells. So it attacks everything. And that causes inflammation. Pain. Damage. All over my body."

"You don't catch it from someone. It's not contagious. You can't get it from me. It's genetic. You inherit it. From your mom's side or your dad's side. Sometimes it skips generations. Sometimes it skips siblings. Sometimes it shows up randomly. But it's in the family somewhere. In the genes."

"You can still live a healthy lifestyle with lupus. But it requires work. A lot of work. You need a team of doctors. Not just one. A whole team. A family of doctors. Each one managing a different part of the disease. Each one keeping a different organ healthy."

"You need a primary doctor for regular checkups. Blood work. General health. Making sure everything is functioning."

"You need a dermatologist for your skin. Because lupus attacks skin. Causes rashes. Causes dryness. Causes problems. And a dermatologist helps manage that. Keeps your skin as healthy as possible."

"You need a nutritionist for a healthy diet. Because what you eat affects lupus. Certain foods trigger inflammation. Certain foods reduce inflammation. You need to know the difference. You need to eat right. And a nutritionist helps with that."

"You need a kidney specialist. Because lupus loves kidneys. It attacks them. Damages them. And kidney damage is serious. Life-threatening. So you need someone monitoring them. Constantly. Making sure they're still working."

"You need a dentist. Because lupus affects your mouth. Your teeth. Your gums. Causes problems. And oral health affects overall health. So you can't neglect that."

"And most of all, you need a rheumatologist. The king or queen of lupus management. The specialist who understands the disease. Who prescribes the right medications. Who monitors the symptoms. Who adjusts the treatment. Who keeps the lupus stable enough that you can actually live your life. Without a good rheumatologist? You're struggling. With one? You're managing. You're living. You're surviving."

"So that's your family of doctors. And you need all of them. Working together. Keeping you healthy. Keeping lupus under control. That's how you live with this disease. That's how you survive."

And usually, after I explain it like that, people get it. They understand. It's not simple. It's not easy. But it's manageable. With the right team. With the right approach. With the right commitment. You can live with lupus. You can thrive with lupus. It's just work. A lot of work. But it's possible.

Has hiding your condition ever caused problems in a relationship or work?

Well, of course it does and it will.

For one, if you don't tell your employment you have serious health issues dealing with lupus, you might be at work on a very busy important day. And lupus is tricky. You can be doing so well one minute. And out of the blue, it can kick in causing you a lot of pain with difficulty of moving around or even functioning in a normal manner.

And it's the same almost for a relationship with friends or a girlfriend.

If you hide it to a certain degree and one day they want to hang out, or your girlfriend wants to be in a hugging position. And you can't hang out with your buddies and you already made them a promise, especially a music concert and they purchased you a ticket in advance and they can't get a refund.

And when you at a time want to hug your girlfriend and can't do it, she will think otherwise if something is wrong with her.

So you see the picture now? So never be surprised if your guy friends or girlfriend have a problem because there will be a time when it will cause problems.

Hiding lupus caused a lot of problems. Big problems. In relationships. In work. In friendships. In every area of life. Because when you hide something that affects your daily life, people don't understand why you act the way you act. Why you cancel plans. Why you can't do things. Why you're distant sometimes. And they fill in the blanks with their own assumptions. And those assumptions are usually wrong. And usually hurtful.

I remember one time I was working at a barbershop. Busy Saturday. Back-to-back clients. And I was doing fine. Cutting hair. Talking. Laughing. Normal day. And then, out of nowhere, lupus hit. Pain shot through my joints. My hands started hurting. My back started aching. My legs started swelling. And I couldn't move the same way. Couldn't stand as long. Couldn't hold the clippers as steady. And my clients noticed. They asked: "You okay, man? You seem off today." And I said: "Yeah, I'm fine. Just tired." But I wasn't fine. I was in pain. Serious pain. And I was trying to push through it. Trying to finish the day. Trying not to let lupus win.

But my boss noticed too. Pulled me aside. Said: "What's going on? You're moving slow. You're not focused. Clients are waiting. You need to pick it up." And I wanted to tell him. I wanted to say: "I have lupus. I'm in pain. I'm doing the best I can." But I didn't. Because I was scared. Scared he'd fire me. Scared he'd see me as a liability. Scared he'd think I couldn't handle the job. So I just said: "I'm good. I'll pick it up." And I pushed harder. Ignored the pain. Finished the day. But it was hard. Really hard. And it shouldn't have been that hard. If I had just told him. If I had just been honest. He might have understood. Might have let me take a break. Might have adjusted the schedule. But I didn't give him that chance. Because I was hiding.

I had this friend. Let's call him Ike. And Ike was always planning things. Concerts. Games. Trips. And he'd invite me. And I'd say yes. Because I wanted to go. I wanted to be normal. I wanted to hang out. But then the day would come. And lupus would flare up. And I'd have to cancel. Last minute. And Ike would be mad. "Bro, you always do this. You always cancel. What's your problem? Are you avoiding me? Do you not want to hang out anymore?" And I'd make excuses. "Something came up. I'm not feeling well. Maybe next time." But I never explained. Never told him about lupus. Never gave him the real reason. So he thought I was flaking. Thought I was a bad friend. Thought I didn't care. And eventually, he stopped inviting me. Stopped reaching out. Stopped trying. And I lost a friend. Because I was hiding.

I dated a woman once. Before I met my fiancée. And she was great. But I didn't tell her about my lupus. Kept it hidden. And there were days when the pain was bad. Couldn't hold hands. Because my body hurt too much. And she'd ask: "What's wrong? Why are you pulling away? Is something wrong with me? Are you not attracted to me anymore?" And I'd say: "No, it's not you. I'm just tired. I'm just stressed." But it was lupus. It was pain. It was my body betraying me. And she didn't know. So she assumed. Assumed I wasn't into her. Assumed I was losing interest. Assumed the relationship was ending. And eventually, it did end. Because I wasn't honest. Because I was hiding. Because I didn't give her the chance to understand.

So yes, hiding lupus caused problems. Serious problems. In every area of life. And I learned the hard way: hiding doesn't protect you. It isolates you. It pushes people away. It makes things harder. Not easier. Honesty, it's scary. But hiding is worse.

So yes, this is one of the biggest reasons why I've started to be more open about telling people about me having lupus. To avoid future problems. So people who I have a lot going on with will understand my situation. And if I can't be around someone or deal with something that day and time, they will have a better understanding.

What made me finally decide to be more open? Simple. I was tired. Tired of hiding. Tired of making excuses. Tired of losing friendships. Tired of straining relationships. Tired of feeling like I had to pretend to be okay when I wasn't. Tired of carrying the burden alone.

I realized: hiding lupus wasn't protecting me. It was hurting me. It was making my life harder. It was creating problems that didn't need to exist. If people knew, they'd understand. They'd be patient. They'd adjust. They'd support. But if they don't know, they can't do any of that. They just think you're flaky. Or moody. Or distant. Or unreliable. And that's not fair to them. And it's not fair to you.

So I decided: I'm going to start telling people. Not everyone. Not strangers. But people who are in my life. People I interact with regularly. People who need to know. Friends. Coworkers. Romantic partners. Family. I'm going to be honest. I'm going to explain. I'm going to give them the chance to understand. And if they can't handle it, if they walk away, that's okay. At least I know. At least I'm not wasting time on people who can't support me. At least I'm surrounding myself with people who get it. Who accept it. Who work with me. Not against me.

And that decision changed everything. Once I started being open, once I started telling people, once I stopped hiding, life got easier. Not physically. Lupus didn't get better. But emotionally. Relationally. Socially. Life got better. Because I wasn't carrying the secret anymore. I wasn't pretending anymore. I wasn't alone anymore. I had people who knew. Who understood. Who supported. And that made all the difference.

Can I share a time when someone's reaction hurt me?

Well, let me tell you. When I was five years into learning lupus, I remember sitting around some older fellows I looked up to.

I always felt I could learn from their ways. I was always admiring the way these older fellows would get together and get their coffee and sandwiches and sit around and talk and be full of laughter.

Until they all took turns talking about their health issues. And when it was my turn, I mentioned I have lupus.

And the number one guy I looked up to said: "Aww man, you're young. Your life is over for you. The older you get, the more problems you will have. You will never be the same, little man."

And I was shocked and depressed. I didn't even want to sit around them anymore after that comment.

That hurt. More than anything anyone has ever said to me about lupus. Because it came from someone I respected. Someone I looked up to. Someone I thought had wisdom. Someone I thought would encourage me. And instead, he crushed me.

Let me give you the full context. I was five years into learning about lupus. Five years into managing it. Five years into figuring out how to live with it. And I was doing okay. Not great. But okay. I was surviving. I was functioning. I was adjusting. And I thought: Maybe I can do this. Maybe I can live a normal life. Maybe lupus doesn't have to ruin everything.

There was this group of older men who used to meet at a coffee shop. Every Saturday morning. They'd get their coffee. Their sandwiches. And they'd sit around and talk. About life. About sports. About politics. About family. About health. And I loved watching them. Listening to them. Learning from them. They had lived long lives. Had wisdom. Had experience. And I wanted to be like them. I wanted to grow old like them. Still meeting friends. Still laughing. Still enjoying life.

So one day, I joined them. Asked if I could sit. They said yes. And I became part of the group. Youngest one there by far. But they accepted me. Treated me like one of them. And I loved it.

And on this particular Saturday, they were talking about their health. One had diabetes. One had high blood pressure. One had bad knees. One had heart problems. And they were joking about it. Making light of it. Talking about their medications. Their doctors. Their limitations. But also talking about how they were managing. How they were still living. How they weren't letting their health issues stop them.

And then someone asked me: "What about you, young man? You have any health issues?" And I hesitated. Because I hadn't told them yet. But I thought: These are older men. They have health issues too. They'll understand. They'll be supportive. So I said: "Yeah. I have lupus."

And the room went quiet. They all looked at me. And then the man I respected most, the one I looked up to the most, the leader of the group, he shook his head. And he said: "Aww man, you're young. Your life is over for you. The older you get, the more problems you will have. You will never be the same, little man."

And I felt like I'd been punched in the gut. Life is over? Never be the same? That's what he had to say? Not encouragement. Not support. Not "you'll be okay" or "you can manage this" or "I believe in you." Just: Your life is over.

I didn't say anything. I just sat there. In shock. Feeling my hope drain away. Feeling my confidence crumble. Feeling like maybe he was right. Maybe my life was over. Maybe I should just give up now. Save myself the trouble of fighting a losing battle.

I finished my coffee. Made an excuse. Left. And I never went back. Never sat with those men again. Because I couldn't. Not after that. Not after hearing that my life was over from someone I respected. It hurt too much. And it stuck with me. For years. That comment. That judgment. That death sentence. It haunted me.

But eventually, I proved him wrong. I'm still here. Still living. Still thriving. Still fighting. My life isn't over. It's different. It's harder. But it's not over. And I'm glad I didn't listen to him. I'm glad I didn't give up. I'm glad I kept fighting. Because he was wrong. Dead wrong. And I'm living proof.

Conversely, tell you about someone whose reaction was supportive.

It was a friend of a friend whose family was dealing with lupus, living with lupus for 20 years or more.

So when I told him what I was dealing with and suffering from, he said: "Oh, okay. My baby's mother is suffering from lupus."

And so he started telling me everything he does for her when she's going through the motions and side effects with dealing with lupus.

And he said: "Don't worry about it. You'll be okay as long as you do what the doctors tell you."

"And if you need any connection on different rheumatologists, we dealt with a few of them. Most of them good. It's just that we try to keep with a rheumatologist close to our hometown."

I said: "Thank you. I appreciate that."

This reaction was the opposite of the older fellow's reaction. And it came from someone I barely knew. A friend of a friend. Not someone close. Not someone I expected anything from. But he gave me exactly what I needed. Hope. Encouragement. Support. Practical help.

I was at a barbecue. Mutual friend's house. And this guy, let's call him Marsoose, was there. We'd met a few times before. Knew each other casually. But weren't close. And somehow, lupus came up in conversation. Someone asked me how I was doing. And I said: "Dealing with some health stuff. It's called lupus." And Marsoose's eyes lit up. Not in a bad way. But in recognition. Like he knew exactly what I was talking about.

And he said: "Oh, okay. My baby's mother has lupus. She's been dealing with it for 20 years. Maybe more. She's doing alright. Managing it. Living her life." And just hearing that, hearing that someone he knew had lupus and was still living, still functioning, still okay after 20 years, that gave me hope. Because I was still new to it. Still scared. Still worried about the future. And hearing that someone had lived with it for two decades and was still going? That was powerful.

And then he did something I didn't expect. He started sharing practical advice. Not just vague encouragement. But real, actionable information. He told me everything he does for his baby's mother when she's having a flare. How he helps her. What works. What doesn't. What to avoid. What to embrace. He told me about her diet. Her exercise routine. Her medication schedule. Her doctor appointments. Her coping mechanisms. Everything.

And then he said: "Don't worry about it. You'll be okay as long as you do what the doctors tell you. Take your meds. Go to your appointments. Listen to your body. Don't push too hard. Don't give up. You'll be okay." And it was simple. But it was exactly what I needed to hear. Not "your life is over." But "you'll be okay." Not doom and gloom. But hope and possibility.

And then he went further. He offered to connect me with his baby's mother's rheumatologist. Said they'd dealt with a few. Most of them good. And if I needed a recommendation, he'd give it to me. He didn't have to do that. We weren't close. He didn't owe me anything. But he did it anyway. Because he understood. Because he'd seen someone he cared about go through it. And he didn't want me to struggle alone. He wanted to help. And he did.

I took him up on his offer. Got the recommendation. Found a great rheumatologist. One of the best I've ever had. And it all started because of Marsoose. Because he was supportive. Because he shared his experience. Because he cared enough to help a guy he barely knew. That's the kind of reaction that matters. That's the kind of support that saves lives. And I'll never forget it.

How do I handle it when people share negative stories about lupus?

I say to them: "Well, everyone's situation is different. Who knows how a person's living behind closed doors while living with lupus?"

"Were they on drugs? Did they smoke cigarettes? Did they drink a lot of alcohol? Did they take all their medications? Did they take any medications? Did they stay with all their doctor's appointments? Did they listen to their doctors? You just never know."

"But I know I was and will do what I am supposed to do, especially if I care about my life and the people who love me."

"So I just brush off that person's negative stories and keep moving."

People love sharing negative stories about lupus. I don't know why. Maybe they think they're helping. Maybe they think they're preparing you. Maybe they're just making conversation. But it's not helpful. It's harmful. It's scary. It's depressing. And I've learned to shut it down.

Someone will say: "Oh, you have lupus? My cousin had that. She died." Or: "My friend's aunt had lupus. She was in the hospital all the time. So much pain. So much suffering. She couldn't work. Couldn't function. It was terrible." Or: "I saw a documentary about lupus. It destroys your organs. Your kidneys fail. Your heart fails. It's awful."

And they say these things like they're just facts. Like they're just sharing information. But what they're really doing is scaring me. Making me think: Is that my future? Am I going to die? Am I going to be in constant pain? Am I going to lose my organs? Am I going to end up in the hospital unable to function?

And at first, those stories affected me. They scared me. Made me anxious. Made me depressed. Made me think: Maybe I should just give up now. Maybe fighting is pointless. Maybe that's where I'm headed anyway.

But then I realized something: everyone's situation is different. Their story is not my story. Their outcome is not my outcome. Their lupus is not my lupus. And there are so many variables. So many factors. So many choices that affect how lupus plays out.

Were they on drugs? Did they smoke? Did they drink heavily? Did they take their medications? Did they go to their doctor's appointments? Did they listen to their doctors? Did they manage their diet? Did they manage their stress? Did they take care of themselves? Or did they ignore it? Did they give up? Did they stop fighting?

You just never know. You don't know what they were doing behind closed doors. You don't know how they were living. You don't know what choices they were making. So their story might be completely different from yours. Their outcome might be completely different from yours. And you can't let their story become your story.

So now, when people share negative stories, I shut it down. Politely. But firmly. I say: "Well, everyone's situation is different. Who knows how they were living. I'm managing mine. I'm taking care of myself. I'm doing what I'm supposed to do. And I'm going to be okay." And then I change the subject. Or I walk away. Because I'm not going to let their negativity become my reality. I'm not going to let their fear become my fear. I'm fighting my own fight. And I'm going to win. Regardless of what happened to someone else.

Slowly but shortly, as I started getting comfortable with some of the individuals I was dealing with and I know

I'll be dealing with for most of my life journey, I explained to them what I was living with. Wow, they had no idea. They were in a state of shock.

Most individuals said: "But if you didn't tell us, we would have never known." Most others said: "You didn't look like you have something serious like lupus."

Some individuals said: "How are you keeping yourself up like the way you are and not showing any signs?"

And yes, most people said what I didn't want to hear. That's why I tried not to tell anyone about what I was dealing with. Because a lot of times, they will tell me about a cousin of theirs or a friend of theirs or a celebrity who passed away from lupus.

I didn't need no negative news or reminding messages like that to linger on my mind all day. Not saying it didn't anyway.

But this is why I spend most of my time trying to make me happy. God knows I was always trying to make others happy first and putting myself last.

And when it was time to do something for me, I was too burnt out. It was like I just kept putting life on hold until I got finished fulfilling someone else's mission for that time, that day.

And yes, that also started to wear and tear on me. So I knew I just had to stop putting myself last, no matter what.

Even when it came to the most close and precious ones in my life, especially for the individuals who knew all about what I was going through and dealing with, they just didn't care. They wanted what they wanted and that was it. Like no type of filter or remorse.

And until this day, it's the same routine. No one cares who you would think would care. But ones you least expect not to really care is the ones that care. How shocked I am still to this day.

So what is good for the ones who don't see it's a problem, I myself had to be the same just to get through some of the times I needed the most with myself.

Well, do I wish people would understand about living with an invisible illness?

I wish they would understand that if you can't really see it, that it can be controlled, it's definitely worth keeping moving on with your life and future plans.

And you don't have to be afraid of it. Because if you have an invisible illness, in some form or fashion, you were blessed with this invisible disease to probably change your lifestyle or to take life seriously with yourself anyway.

What I wish people understood about invisible illness is this: Just because you can't see it doesn't mean it's not real. Just because I look okay doesn't mean I am okay. Just because I'm functioning doesn't mean I'm not struggling. Just because I'm smiling doesn't mean I'm not in pain.

Lupus is invisible most of the time. You can't see the inflammation. You can't see the joint pain. You can't see the fatigue. You can't see the organ damage. You can't see the immune system attacking itself. All you see is me. Standing there. Looking normal. Acting normal. And you assume I'm fine. But I'm not. I'm just really good at hiding it.

And I wish people understood: when I cancel plans last minute, it's not because I don't want to see you. It's because my body won't let me. When I'm quiet or distant, it's not because I'm mad at you. It's because I'm in pain and trying to manage it. When I say I'm tired, I don't mean I didn't sleep well. I mean my whole body is exhausted from fighting itself. When I say I can't do something, I'm not being lazy. I'm being realistic about my limitations.

I wish people understood: living with an invisible illness is lonely. Because people can't see what you're going through. They can't understand. They think you're exaggerating. Or faking. Or being dramatic. Or looking for attention. But you're not. You're just trying to survive. You're just trying to live. You're just trying to function despite your body working against you.

I wish people understood: we're not asking for pity. We're not asking for special treatment. We're just asking for understanding. For patience. For compassion. For the benefit of the doubt. For the recognition that just because you can't see our illness doesn't mean it's not affecting every aspect of our lives.

And I wish people understood: having an invisible illness doesn't mean giving up on life. It doesn't mean your life is over. It doesn't mean you can't have dreams. Can't have goals. Can't have a future. It just means you have to adapt. You have to be more careful. You have to manage yourself better. You have to work harder to maintain what others take for granted. But you can still live. You can still thrive. You can still be happy. Your illness is invisible. But so is your strength. And your strength is greater than your illness. That's what I wish people understood.

Chapter 18
The Affections of a Favorite Pet

I didn't know how long I was going to keep up a healthy routine like exercises and eating the right foods or just to keep myself moving so that I don't sit around feeling sorry for myself, being in a deep depressed mood.

So even though I was in a relationship, I still felt like I was missing something else.

I mean, being in a relationship, you know you both have a job to do together to keep the relationship together. And you both got to take time apart for other individuals who are in our lives and other projects we are working on in our lives for our future together and for ourselves.

Like going to work for a couple of hours, going to school to achieve some type of degree or trade. And but not least, family and friends we will go visit by ourselves.

And yes, we both need time for ourselves like some me time. Time to take a moment to pamper ourselves, treat ourselves with something special. So that we can meditate, concentrate, and focus on some of the goals we are trying to accomplish, like financial freedom.

So when I could not keep up with my spouse because the lupus would be very active on some days, I needed something to keep to my side and hold on to if my spouse was with me still at that moment of going through a depressed mood and pain.

Let me explain something about living with lupus in a relationship. Even the best relationship. Even with the most supportive partner. There are still moments when you're alone. Not physically alone. But emotionally alone. Mentally alone. In your pain alone.

Because your partner has a life. They have work. They have responsibilities. They have family. They have friends. They have their own needs. Their own goals. Their own dreams. And that's normal. That's healthy. That's how relationships should be. You can't expect one person to be everything for you. To be with you every single moment. To meet every single need. That's not fair to them. And it's not realistic.

But when lupus is active, when the pain is bad, when you're going through a depressed mood, when you're struggling, you need something. Someone. A presence. A companion. Someone constant. Someone who doesn't have to leave for work. Someone that doesn't have other obligations. Someone that's just there. Always. No matter what.

And that's what I was missing. That constant presence. That unconditional companionship. Something to keep me moving when I didn't feel like moving. Something to keep me focused when all I wanted to do was give up.

Something to remind me that I'm not alone even when my fiancée had to be somewhere else.

So I decided to adopt a pet. A dog. Because I'd heard that dogs help with depression. With anxiety. With loneliness. With healing. And I needed all of that. I needed help. And I thought that maybe a dog can give me what I'm missing. Maybe a dog can fill that void. Maybe a dog can be that constant presence I need to keep going.

I had no idea how right I was. I had no idea that this decision would change my life. I had no idea that God was about to send me an angel in the form of a brown pitbull puppy. I had no idea that Brown Sugar was about to become more than just a pet. She was about to become my healer. My companion. My reason to keep fighting. My guardian angel.

I decided to adopt my favorite pet. I adopted a puppy and named her Brown Sugar.

Brown Sugar was a brown female blue nose pitbull. She was a special gift from God.

I purchased her from some street guys who had an abandoned house where they would breed dogs to sell as a business.

My fiancée always told me stories about a dog she used to have when she was younger. And her brother and father gave him away to some people they knew. So she said she was so hurt that she cried for some time. So that story stuck with me for a while.

So once I found out who was selling puppies, I went and purchased one.

But the way it went about was the mother and father were brown. And all the other puppies were black with a white stripe down their neck. And Brown Sugar was hiding in the corner of the room they had all the puppies in.

Let me describe Brown Sugar in detail. Because she was beautiful. Unique. One of a kind.

She was a brown female blue nosed pitbull. And when I say brown, I mean a light tan brownish color. With a white stripe going down from her neck to her chest. Just like her mom and dad. That's what made her special. That's what made her stand out.

Because all her siblings came out black. All of them. Black with a white stripe on the neck. But Brown Sugar? She came out looking exactly like her parents. The only one. The special one. The chosen one.

Her face had this look. This expression. A little frown. Like she was always thinking. Always observing. Always serious. But when she was happy, when she smiled, her whole face would light up. Her eyes would sparkle. And you could feel the love radiating from her.

Well and like I said she was a blue nose pit. That's the pitbull trait. And it made her look distinguished. Regal. Like royalty. And as she grew, she became strong. Muscular. Powerful. But gentle. So gentle. Especially with me. Especially when I was in pain.

Her coat was smooth. Shiny. Beautiful. And she loved being petted. Loved being brushed. Would sit there for hours just letting you love on her. And she'd lean into you. Put her full weight on you. Like she was trying to hug you back. Like she was saying: I love you, too.

That was Brown Sugar. My special gift from God. My angel.

When I went to adopt her from the abandoned trap house, and as I was trying to pick out a puppy, there were many. And they all had a look of how this certain type of breed should look like.

But there was one who stood out because she was the smallest in size from all the rest. And how she stood alone from the rest of the pack. She was shivering and scared, looking up, alone in the corner of the room.

I just knew she was special because out of eight puppies, she was the only one who came out looking like the mother and father.

And like I said, she was living in an unfit abandoned house with other dogs that wasn't being properly taken care of. And Brown Sugar was the smallest puppy. She was scared. She was a little dirty. Definitely hungry.

Let me tell you about that day. The day I met Brown Sugar. The day God put her in my path. The day my life changed. I've been living with lupus for quite a while now. I got diagnosed with lupus in my 20s. Managing it. Surviving it. But struggling with it. Emotionally. Mentally. I needed something. And my fiancée kept telling me about this dog she had when she was younger. How much she loved that dog. How hurt she was when her brother and father gave him away. How she cried for weeks. And that story stuck with me. I thought: Maybe I can get her a dog. Replace the one she lost. Make her happy. And maybe it'll help me too.

So I started asking around. Who has puppies? Who's selling dogs? And someone told me about these street guys who breed pitbulls in an abandoned house. Not the best situation. Not the most ethical. But I didn't care at the time. I just wanted a dog.

So I went to this abandoned house. And it was rough. Definitely not fit for animals. Not fit for people. But there they were. The mother dog. The father dog. And about eight puppies. All running around. Playing. Wrestling. Cute. Energetic. Healthy-looking.

Except one.

In the corner of the room, all by herself, was the smallest puppy. Brown. While all her siblings were black. Shivering. Scared. She was a little dirty. Hungry. Neglected. And she just sat there. Looking up at me. With these big, sad eyes. Like she was saying: please, take me. Get me out of here.

And I looked at all the other puppies. The black ones. The healthy ones. The ones running around. And I asked the guys: "Can I buy one of the black and white puppies?" And they kept telling me no. Because people had already put money down on them. They were reserved. Sold. Spoken for.

And I offered more money. Kept begging. "Please, I'll pay extra. Just let me have one of the black ones." And they just were not agreeing. They said no. Firm. Final.

So I looked back at the brown puppy in the corner. The one nobody wanted. The one nobody reserved. The one sitting there alone. Scared. And something in me said you know what, I believe God wants you to have that one. That's your dog. That's who you're supposed to take home. I said yeah, I guess it was meant to be this brown one, because it's no way in the world somebody that's in this type of business and living like this will turn down some extra money.

And I said, "Okay, I'll take her." And I purchased Brown Sugar. Paid for her. Picked her up. And brought her home.

And I am so glad I did. Because she turned out to be the best support, healing power, therapy dog I've ever had. She wasn't a mistake. She wasn't my choice. She was God's choice. God put her in that corner. God made sure the black puppies were reserved. God made sure she was saved for me. Because she was meant for me. And I was meant for her.

And that's another thing that drew me to say that I'll buy her. Because she had a special type of look and frown on her face. And she was the only one who looked like the mom and dad dog. That told me she's different. She's special. She's the one.

After a while, as a puppy, she used to watch me moan when in pain, watch me bandage up both my legs and take my medications.

She watched me like she knew what was going on with me. Like she was supposed to be here. Or sent by God as my guardian angel.

As I went through all the difficult times with lupus, always at the same time taking medications and always at the same time cleaning and changing the wrapping on the wounds on my legs, Brown Sugar had been watching me at all times.

Brown Sugar learned my routine faster than I expected. It just didn't seem possible for a puppy. It was like she understood. Like she knew. Like God gave her special knowledge about what I was going through. About what I needed. About how to help me.

Every morning, I'd wake up. And the first thing I'd do is check my legs. See how the wounds looked. See if they were healing. See if they were infected. See if they leaked overnight. And Brown Sugar would be right there. Sitting next to the bed. Watching. Waiting. Like she knew what was coming next.

Then I'd get my supplies. The gauze. The tape. The ointment. The bandages. And I'd sit on the edge of the bed or on the couch. And I'd start cleaning the wounds. And it hurt. Every time. No matter how gentle I was. No matter how careful. It hurt. And I'd moan. Wince. Sometimes cry. From the pain. From the frustration. From the exhaustion of dealing with this every single day.

And Brown Sugar would watch. Intently. Like she was studying. Like she was learning. Like she was memorizing every step. Every product. Every motion. She'd tilt her head. Observe. Take it all in. And she never left. Never got distracted. Never wandered off. She just watched. Like it was her job. Like she was my nurse in training.

Then I'd take my medications. Pull out the pill bottles. Line them up. Count them out. Take them one by one with water. And Brown Sugar would watch that too. She'd sniff the bottles. Memorize the routine. Learn the schedule. And after a while, she started anticipating it. She'd bring me the bag with my medications before I even asked. Before I even remembered. Like she had an internal clock. Like she knew it was time.

It was incredible. Unbelievable. Almost supernatural. How could a dog know this? How could a puppy understand this? How could she learn this so quickly? Unless God taught her. Unless God sent her specifically to help me. Unless she was more than just a dog. Unless she was an angel. A guardian. A gift from heaven.

And I started thinking, did Brown Sugar have my grandmother inside of her? Or was it someone who cared about me many years ago that passed away and came back as a female dog? Or did God just put this dog in my life to help me with lupus?

I didn't know the answer. But I did know that Brown Sugar was special. She was different. She was sent. And I was blessed to have her.

When I used to come home after running around, the first thing Brown Sugar would do was go grab my bag that had my medications inside and drag it to me.

And the first time she ever did that, I was amazed. I was in shock.

I couldn't stop thinking about when I was younger, how I used to hear adults talking about how some people that pass away get reincarnated.

So I started thinking: Did Brown Sugar have my grandmother inside of her spiritually? Or was it someone who cared about me many years ago that passed away and came back as a female dog?

Or did God just put this dog in my life to help me with lupus?

It kept me thinking about every move Brown Sugar did around me that related to what a human would do.

And I knew there wasn't a mistake that she was in both my fiancée and I's life.

The medication bag moment. That was the moment I knew for certain that Brown Sugar was sent by God. Because what she did was impossible. Unexplainable. Unless she had divine knowledge.

I'd come home from running errands. Or from hanging out. Or from a doctor's appointment. And I'd be tired. Exhausted. In pain. And I'd sit on the couch. And before I could even catch my breath, Brown Sugar would run to where I kept my medication bag. Grab it with her mouth. Drag it across the floor. And bring it to me. Drop it at my feet. Then sit there. Looking at me. Like she was saying: "Take your meds. It's time. Don't forget."

The first time she did it, I was in shock. I thought it was a coincidence. Maybe she just liked carrying things. Maybe she was playing. But then she did it again. And again. And again. Every single time I came home. Without fail. Without being trained. Without being told. She just knew.

And I started thinking, how does she know? How does she know that bag has my medications? How does she know I need to take them? How does she know the schedule? Dogs are smart. But this? This is beyond smart. This is supernatural. This is divine.

And that's when I started wondering about reincarnation. I'd heard about it when I was younger. Adults talking. Saying that people who pass away can come back. In different forms. As different beings. And I would wonder if that was possible. Could my grandmother be in Brown Sugar? Could someone I loved who died be guiding this dog? Teaching her? Using her to help me?

I don't know if reincarnation is real. I don't know if that's how it works. But I know this: Brown Sugar acted like a human. Thought like a human. Cared like a human. She anticipated my needs. Remembered my routines. Helped me in ways that seemed impossible for a dog. And that made me believe: She's not just a dog. She's more. She's an angel. She's a blessing. She's a gift from God.

And every move she made around me confirmed it. The way she'd lay her head on my lap when I was sad. The way she'd nudge my hand when I was staring into space, lost in depression. The way she'd bark to wake me from nightmares. The way she'd refuse to leave my side when I was sick. All of it. Human-like. Intentional. Loving. Divine.

She wasn't a mistake. She was meant to be in our lives. Mine and my fiancée's. God knew I needed her. God knew she could help me in ways that medicine couldn't. In ways that doctors couldn't. In ways that even my fiancée couldn't. Because Brown Sugar had something special. Something supernatural. Something sent from heaven. And I was blessed to receive it.

Once she got used to me and my fiancée, I tell you, it was like raising a spoiled child.

She used to get into everything that would make a mess in the house. And she had some type of personality with herself. If she was upset with you, she would let you know.

If I was to not let her have her way with me, she would sit around looking at what I like. And when I wasn't around, she would get it and chew it up, destroying it totally.

Like my favorite sneaker or shoes, the TV remote, the cord to my blender or hair clippers.

But when it came to my fiancée making her upset, she wouldn't chew up her favorite stuff. But since my fiancée likes kissing on her, when my fiancée tried to kiss Brown Sugar before going to work, Brown Sugar would turn away, letting her know she was upset.

Brown Sugar was something else, I tell you. One of a kind.

Brown Sugar had a personality. A big personality. She wasn't just a dog who did what you told her. She had opinions. She had feelings. She had preferences. And if you crossed her, she'd let you know. In the most creative, vindictive ways possible.

She was spoiled. We admit it. We spoiled her. Because she was our baby. Our child. Our angel. So we gave her everything. Toys, her favorite treats. Whatever she wanted. And she knew it. She knew she was the princess of the house. And she acted like it.

But if you made her mad? If you didn't give her what she wanted? If you told her no? She'd get revenge. And it was calculated. Intentional. Smart.

If I made her upset, she wouldn't attack me. She wouldn't bark at me. She wouldn't ignore me. Instead, she'd study. She'd observe. She'd figure out what I loved most. What I used most around the house. What I'd miss if it was gone. And then, when I wasn't looking, when I left the room, when I went to work, she'd destroy it.

My favorite sneakers? Chewed to pieces. The TV remote? Destroyed. The cord to my blender? Severed. The cord to my hair clippers? Gone. And she'd do it strategically. She'd wait until I was gone. Then she'd find the item. Bring it under the bed with her. And methodically chew it to bits. I guess that was her way of getting revenge, and I used to say to myself okay, so that's how you let me know you upset with me.

And the crazy part? She knew what she did. When I'd come home and find my stuff destroyed, she will find a place to hide in the house.

But with my fiancée? It was different. Brown Sugar loved my fiancée. Adored her. So when my fiancée made her upset, Brown Sugar wouldn't destroy her stuff. She had a different method. A gentler method. But equally effective; the silent treatment.

My fiancée loves kissing Brown Sugar. All the time. On the head. On the face. Constantly. And Brown Sugar usually loved it. Would lean into it. Would lick her back. But if my fiancée had made her upset? If she rubbed her the wrong way. Like if she'd told Brown Sugar no about something she wanted. Then when my fiancée tried to kiss her before going to work, Brown Sugar would turn her head. Refuse the kiss. Pull away. And my fiancée would be devastated. "Brown Sugar, I'm sorry! Come on, give me a kiss!" And Brown Sugar would just sit there. Wouldn't move. Until she was ready to forgive. Until she decided my fiancée had learned her lesson.

That was Brown Sugar. Spoiled. Smart. Vengeful. But also loving. Loyal. Devoted. She had a personality. A sense of humor. A sense of justice. And we loved her for it. All of it. Even when she destroyed our stuff. Even when she refused our kisses. Because that's what made her special. That's what made her Brown Sugar. That's what made her one of a kind.

And when I used to cry myself to sleep because I was in too much pain, Brown Sugar would get in bed, lying next to my side, licking my face or my wounds on my legs, trying to bring me comfort, trying to heal me, trying to help in every way she can.

Brown Sugar would lick my wounds when I leave the wrappings off my legs to get fresh air at some times.

She would lick my wounds for twenty to thirty minutes, easing my pain and suffering I was going through at that moment.

And I would let her do this for me so often.

And my wounds used to heal quickly, then they usually would. Most of the times it takes about four to six months or even close to a year at that time, earlier in the years of dealing with the wounds.

Well, Brown Sugar used to lick on my wounds like every other day. My wounds' process of closing up would start very quickly.

And the wound clinic used to be like: "Wow, good progress we are doing, Johnny. Keep up the good work!"

But they didn't know Brown Sugar was giving them some help also with the healing process.

This is the part that sounds crazy. The part that people don't believe. The part that doctors would never accept. But it's true. It happened. And I witnessed it. Brown Sugar healed my wounds. Literally. Physically. With her saliva. With her tongue. With her love.

Here's how it worked: When I had open wounds on my legs from the varicose veins bursting, from the lupus attacking my skin, I'd have to keep them wrapped most of the time. Bandaged. Protected. But sometimes, I'd take the wrappings off. To let them air out. To let them breathe. To clean them properly. And during those times, Brown Sugar would come over. Sniff the wounds. Then start licking them.

At first, I'd pull away. I'd think: That's not sanitary. That's not clean. Dogs' mouths have bacteria. This could make it worse. This could cause infection. But Brown Sugar was persistent. She'd keep trying. Keep nudging my leg. Keep licking. Like she was saying: "Trust me. I know what I'm doing. Let me help you."

So eventually, I let her. And she'd lick. For 20 to 30 minutes. Gently. Methodically. Covering every inch of the wound. And as she licked, something amazing happened: the pain would ease. The throbbing would stop. The burning would calm. I don't know if it was her saliva. Or the act of licking. Or the warmth of her tongue. Or the love behind it. But it worked. The pain would lessen. And I'd feel comfort. Relief. And a sense of peace.

And over time, I noticed: my wounds healed faster when Brown Sugar licked them. Significantly faster. Wounds that usually took four to six months to close? They'd close in two or three. Wounds that took close to a year? They'd heal in six months. And the wound clinic noticed too. They'd say: "Wow, good progress we're doing, Johnny. Keep up the good work!" And I'd smile. Because then I'll tell them that my dog is helping you guys. Soon you guys will have to give her a job. They will smile and be like oh wow really?

And I believe it. I believe dog saliva has healing properties. I've heard stories. Read articles. About how dogs' saliva has enzymes. Antibacterial properties. Things that promote healing. That kill infection. That speed recovery. And I experienced it. Firsthand. My wounds healed faster. Cleaner. Better. Because of Brown Sugar alongside the wound clinic.

But it wasn't just the physical healing. It was the emotional healing too. When I was in pain, when I was crying, when I was ready to give up, Brown Sugar would climb into bed. Lay next to me. Put her head on my chest. Lick my face. Lick my wounds. And remind me that I was not alone and that she was there. We're in this together. And that emotional support? That unconditional love? That healed me too. Healed my spirit. Healed my mind. Healed my hope.

Brown Sugar didn't just ease my pain. She healed me. In every way possible. And I'm forever grateful.

I can share specific stories of times when Brown Sugar knew I was in pain.

Brown Sugar could always sense when I was in pain because she would always stay by my side, not letting me out of her sight.

When my legs would be leaking pus or my legs were carrying a smell or when Brown Sugar didn't see me do my wrapping routine that I usually do every morning and night.

She would take her nose and tap on my legs where the wounds were, like she was telling me: "It's time to clean your legs. What are you doing?"

So I'd tell her: "I'm sorry, baby girl. I am in too much pain to even change the wrappings right now." I'd tell her: "Later, okay? Come lay next to me in bed."

And Brown Sugar would do just that. And her body heat would help me with some comfort, making the pain ease up.

Let me share specific stories. Times when Brown Sugar knew I was in pain. Times when she helped me. Times when she saved me.

One morning, I woke up in excruciating pain. My legs were throbbing. Leaking. Smelling. I knew I needed to change the wrappings. Clean the wounds. Apply fresh bandages. But I couldn't. The pain was too much. I could barely move. So I just lay there. In bed. Trying to breathe through it. Trying to wait for it to pass.

And Brown Sugar noticed. She came into the bedroom. Jumped on the bed. Sniffed my legs. And she knew something was wrong. She could smell it. The infection. The pus. The decay. And she took her nose and tapped on my legs. Right where the wounds were. Gently. But firmly. Like she was saying: "Dad. You need to take care of this. You need to clean this. What are you doing?"

And I looked at her. And I said: "I'm sorry, baby girl. I am in too much pain to even change the wrappings right now. Later, okay? Come lay next to me in bed." And she did. She climbed up. Laid next to me. Put her body against mine. And her body heat, her warmth, her presence, it helped. The pain eased. Not completely. But enough. Enough to breathe. Enough to rest. Enough to get through that moment.

And later, when I finally had the strength, I changed the wrappings. Cleaned the wounds. And Brown Sugar sat there. Watching. Making sure I did it right. Making sure I took care of myself. Because she cared. Because she knew. Because she was my guardian.

There were times I'd have coughing attacks in my sleep. Or nightmares. Bad ones. The kind where you feel like you're drowning. Like you can't breathe. Like something's on top of you. Holding you down. People call it sleep paralysis. Or "the witch on your back." Whatever it is, it's terrifying. You try to scream. But no sound comes out. You try to move. But you can't. You're trapped. Helpless. Suffocating.

And Brown Sugar would wake me up. She'd jump on the bed. Lick my face. Bark. Loud. Aggressive. Not at me. But at whatever was attacking me. At the evil. At the nightmare. At the witch. And her barking would break through. Would pull me out. Would save me. And I'd wake up. Gasping. Sweating. Shaking. But alive. Awake. Safe. Because of Brown Sugar.

And this happened multiple times. To me. To my fiancée. And every time, Brown Sugar was there. Protecting us. Saving us. Fighting off whatever spiritual attack was happening. She wasn't just a dog. She was a warrior. A guardian angel. Sent by God to watch over us both.

When I was having bad flares, when the lupus was active, when I was in so much pain I couldn't function, Brown Sugar would not leave my side. She'd follow me from room to room. Sit outside the bathroom door. Lay next to the couch where I was resting. Refuse to eat until I ate. Refuse to go outside until I moved. She kept watch. Constant. Vigilant. Like she was my nurse. My protector. My companion.

And her presence helped. More than medicine. More than doctors. More than anything. Because she reminded me that I'm not alone. Someone cares. Someone's here. Someone's fighting with me. And that gave me strength. That gave me hope. That gave me the will to keep going.

That was Brown Sugar. She knew when I was in pain. She sensed it. She responded to it. She helped ease it. And I'll never forget that. Never stop being grateful for that. Never stop missing the kisses of Brown Sugar.

She just brought too much life into my fiancée and I's life.

I didn't care about what was going on in the world or what we were doing at sometimes, as long as Brown Sugar was happy.

I mean, I can write a book on everything she did to let us know she's a God special dog. She was put in our lives to watch over us.

Brown Sugar kept us in shape, no matter how tired we were, no matter what type of weather we were having in the winter.

No matter if it was the rain, below twenty degrees with thick ice all over the ground, the lake frozen, your skin turning blue within 15 minutes of being outside.

Brown Sugar wanted to be outside with us and made sure we all go out for our daily walk around the park.

Brown Sugar brought so much life into our lives. She changed everything. She made us better. Healthier. Happier. More active. More alive.

Before Brown Sugar, I'd make excuses. "It's too cold. It's raining. I'm too tired. I'm in too much pain. I'll walk tomorrow." And tomorrow never came. I'd stay inside. Sit on the couch. Be depressed. Be inactive. And my health would suffer. My lupus would get worse. My joints would stiffen. My weight would increase. My mood would plummet. All because I wasn't moving.

But Brown Sugar? She didn't accept excuses. She didn't care about the weather. She didn't care about my pain. She cared about one thing: that we did our daily walk. And she made sure it happened. Every single day. No matter what.

Every morning, she'd grab her leash. Bring it to me. Drop it at my feet. Sit there. Staring. Waiting. Like: "It's time. Let's go. No excuses." And if I ignored her, she'd nudge me. Bark. Bring the leash again. Until I got up.

Until I put my shoes on. Until I took her out and made sure we all got out of the house for that walk.

And it didn't matter what the weather was. Rain? She wanted to walk. Snow? She wanted to walk. Twenty degrees below zero? She wanted to walk. Thick ice all over the ground? She wanted to walk. The lake frozen solid? She wanted to walk.

And we'd go. Because we couldn't say no to her. Because she needed it. Because we knew it was good for us. Even when it was hard. Even when it hurt. Even when we didn't want to. We'd bundle up. Put on our coats. Our gloves. Our hats. And we'd walk. Around the park. In the freezing cold. In the rain. In the snow. And Brown Sugar would be so happy. Running. Playing. Enjoying every second. And her joy was contagious. We'd start to enjoy it too. Start to feel the benefits. The fresh air. The movement. The exercise. The life.

And I realized: Brown Sugar was keeping us alive. Not just figuratively. But literally. She was forcing us to move. To exercise. To get outside. To stay active. And that helped my lupus. Helped my joints. Helped my mood. Helped my health. She was my personal trainer. My motivator. My reason to keep moving. And I needed that. More than I knew.

Brown Sugar kept us in shape. No matter how tired we were. No matter what the weather was. She made sure we went out for our daily walk. Every single day. And I'm better for it. Healthier for it. Stronger for it. All because of her.

So you know we did have Brown Sugar for quite a while.

Me and my fiancée had Brown Sugar for about sixteen years. And Brown Sugar passed away from a cancerous tumor.

Sixteen years. That's how long I had Brown Sugar. Sixteen beautiful, blessed, life-changing years. From the time I was twenty-eight until I was forty-four. Through my thirties and into my forties. Through the hardest years of living with lupus. Through flares. Through hospitalizations. Through depression. Through pain. Through it all, Brown Sugar was there. By my side. Every single day. For sixteen years.

And those sixteen years were the best years of my life. Not because lupus got better. It didn't. Not because life got easier. It didn't. But because I had Brown Sugar. And she made everything bearable. Manageable. Survivable. She gave me a reason to get up every morning. A reason to keep fighting. A reason to smile even when I wanted to cry. She was my constant. My rock. My angel.

But nothing lasts forever. Not even angels. And eventually, it was time for Brown Sugar to go home. Back to God. Back to heaven. Where she belonged.

It started with a tumor. We noticed it first. A lump. On her side. Small at first. We thought maybe it was nothing. Maybe it was benign. Maybe it would go away. But it didn't. It grew. Slowly. Then faster. And we took her to the vet. And they did tests. Scans. Biopsies. And the diagnosis came back: cancer. Aggressive cancer. Spreading. Terminal.

And our world shattered. Our hearts broke. How could this happen? To Brown Sugar? To our angel? To the dog who saved our lives? It wasn't fair. It wasn't right. We prayed. We cried. We begged God: Please. Not yet. We need more time. Don't take her yet.

But God had other plans. Brown Sugar had completed her mission. She had healed me. Helped me. Loved me. For sixteen years. And now, it was time for her to rest. Time for her to go home. Time for her to return to the God who sent her. I believe the year was 2018 when we lost our Brown Sugar.

Well, she started to go through the moments of transitioning. She wasn't responding when we called her. She started falling every so often into her stoop. She was walking very slowly and getting tired very quickly.

We took Brown Sugar to the vet hospital, hoping they could save her. It was on July 3rd, 2018.

And the vet told us: "She can't be saved. Please let us put her to sleep."

We cried and said: "No, no."

And we took her back home with us. And we said we will let it play out in our home, praying and wishing for a miracle from God.

So she lasted overnight. But it's like she was really starting to suffer.

So we picked her up and rushed her back to the vet hospital. And then the people came out of the truck with a stretcher and took her in to put her to sleep.

But when they grabbed her from the truck, I was next to them. And Brown Sugar took her paws and gripped one of my legs, like she was saying: "I love you. Please don't let them take me."

The experience of seeing this happen took part of my life away with her.

And it still has a big, big effect on me and my fiancée.

July 3rd, 2018. That's the day our world started falling apart. That's the day we knew we were losing her. That's the day we took Brown Sugar to the vet hospital, hoping they could save her. Hoping for a miracle. Hoping for more time.

But they couldn't save her. The vet looked at us with sad eyes. Compassionate eyes. And said: "She can't be saved. The cancer has spread too much. She's in pain. She's suffering. The kindest thing you can do is let us put her to sleep. Let her go peacefully. Without pain. With dignity."

And we cried. We sobbed. We said: "No, no. There has to be something. There has to be a way. Please. Try something. Anything. We can't lose her. Not yet.

Please." But the vet shook his head. "I'm sorry. There's nothing more we can do. It's time."

But we couldn't accept it. We couldn't let go. So we took her back home. We said: "We'll let it play out at home. We'll pray. We'll believe for a miracle. God can heal her. God can save her. We just need to have faith."

So we brought her home. Set her up in the living room. Made her comfortable. Gave her water. Her favorite treats. And we prayed. All night. We stayed up with her. Watching her. Hoping. Believing.

But by morning, we knew. She was suffering. Really suffering. She couldn't stand. Couldn't eat. Couldn't drink. Could barely breathe. And we realized that we were being selfish. We're keeping her here for us. Not for her. She's ready to go. She wants to go. We have to let her go.

So on July 4th, 2018, we picked her up. Wrapped her in her favorite blanket. And rushed her back to the vet hospital. And they were ready. They had a stretcher. They came out to the truck. And they reached in to get her.

And that's when it happened. The moment that will haunt me forever. Brown Sugar, weak as she was, in pain as she was, dying as she was, she took her paws and gripped my leg. Held on. Tight. And looked at me. With those eyes. Those beautiful, loving, trusting eyes. And I knew what she was saying: "I love you. Please don't let them take me. I don't want to go. I want to stay with you."

And I broke. Completely. I cried. I sobbed. I wanted to pull her back. Keep her. Never let go. But I knew I had to. I had to be strong for her. I had to let her go. So I pet her head. Kissed her. And whispered: "I love you too, baby girl. So much. Thank you. Thank you for everything. For sixteen years. For healing me. For loving me. For being my angel. Go home now. Go to God. Go to heaven. It's okay. I'll see you again. I promise."

And they took her. And I watched them carry her inside. And I never saw her alive again. They put her to sleep. Peacefully. Painlessly. And she was gone. My Brown Sugar. My angel. My healer. Gone.

And as I'm writing this now, tears are coming down my face. A chill is running through my body. Because it still hurts. It still affects me. Deeply. Profoundly. It's been years. But the pain hasn't lessened. The loss hasn't diminished. I still miss her. Every single day. And I always will. Yes everyone who's reading my story I can't fully describe the pain of losing something precious as Brown Sugar. And I mean I cried.

I cried for months, non-stop. We had her cremated and still have her ashes. And all her toys. And a bag full of her dead doggy hair.

So at some times when I am alone, I open up the bag and smell her scent.

And I smell her doggy clothes we used to put on her.

Every morning before I start anything, I go into my guest room where I have a shrine and all her pictures. I pick up this one picture and kiss it: "Good morning," like she was still here with us. Still alive running around the house waiting for us to take her outside, we still feel her presence very strongly around the house.

It's what I used to do when she was living. I'd get up and hug and give her a kiss.

And this is how I cope with the loss of Brown Sugar until this very day.

And Brown Sugar has passed away, going on five years now.

I have many, many pictures and videos of her.

How do I cope? Not well. Not easily. Not without pain. But I cope. Day by day. Memory by memory. Ritual by ritual.

After she passed, we had her cremated. We couldn't bury her. Couldn't leave her in the ground. We needed her close. So we had her cremated. And we brought her ashes home. In a beautiful urn. And we placed it in the guest room. On a shelf. Surrounded by her pictures. Her collar. Her favorite toys. Like a shrine. A memorial. A sacred space where we can go to be close to her.

And I kept everything. Everything. Her toys. Her blankets. Her clothes we used to put on her. I didn't wash them. But kept them. Because they still smell like her. And when I'm missing her, when the pain is too much, I pull out one of her sweaters. And I smell it. And for a moment, she's back. For a moment, I can feel her. Sense her. Remember her. And it helps. Not much. But a little.

And she still comes to me. In my dreams. I see her. Running. Playing. Licking my face. Bringing me my medication bag. Lying next to me. And I wake up. And for a split second, I forget. I think she's still here. And then reality hits. And I remember. She's gone. But those dreams? They're a gift. They're God letting me see her again. Letting me feel her again. Letting me know that she's okay. She's in heaven. She's happy. She's waiting for me.

That's how I cope. It's not perfect. It's not complete. But it's all I have. And it's enough. Until I see her again. In heaven. Where we'll be reunited. Where I'll hug her again. Kiss her again. Thank her again. For sixteen beautiful years. For being my angel. For saving my life.

No way. No, I am not ready still. After all this time, not ready to replace Brown Sugar.

Would I adopt another pet?

At this time, I will not. It's still hurting till this day. It's been five years now.

We thought about it. We talked about it. We had people whose dogs had puppies try to give us puppies. And we turned them down.

Just can't take a loss of something that precious again in my life right now.

No. Nothing has filled that void. No one has replaced Brown Sugar. And I don't think anything or anyone ever will. Because she wasn't just a pet. She was my angel. My healer. My companion. My purpose. You don't replace that. You can't replace that.

People ask us all the time: "When are you getting another dog? You should get a puppy. It'll help you heal. It'll help you move on." And I know they mean well. I know they're trying to help. But they don't understand. Getting another dog isn't moving on. It's not healing. It's replacing. And I can't replace Brown Sugar. I won't replace Brown Sugar.

We've thought about it. Many times. We've talked about it. Debated it. My fiancée says: "Maybe it would help. Maybe a puppy would bring life back into the house. Maybe it would give us something to focus on."

And part of me agrees. Part of me thinks that maybe she's right. Maybe a new dog would help. Maybe it would ease the pain.

But then I think about Brown Sugar. About how special she was. About how she knew me. Understood me. Helped me. Healed me. And I think: another dog won't do that. Another dog won't be her. Another dog will just remind me of what I lost. And I can't handle that. Not yet. Maybe not ever.

And people have tried to give us puppies. Friends whose dogs had litters. They'd say: "We have puppies. We'll give you one. Free. Please. You need a dog. You love dogs." And we'd turn them down. Politely. Firmly. "Thank you. But no. We're not ready. We can't. Not yet."

Because we're still hurting. Deeply. Profoundly. It's been four years. Almost five. And it feels like yesterday. The pain hasn't lessened. The loss hasn't diminished. I still cry. I still miss her. I still feel the void. And bringing another dog into that void? It wouldn't fill it. It would just make it more obvious. More painful. More empty.

So no, I haven't adopted another pet. I won't adopt another pet. Not right now. Not until I'm ready. If I'm ever ready. Because losing Brown Sugar? It took part of my life away. Part of my heart. Part of my soul. And I can't go through that again. I can't love like that again. Only to lose it again. It's too much. Too painful. Too hard.

Maybe one day. Maybe in the future. Maybe when the pain eases. Maybe when I'm stronger. Maybe God will send me another angel. Another Brown Sugar. Another healer. But until then? I'm honoring her memory. Cherishing what we had. And missing her. Every single day.

The most amazing thing Brown Sugar ever did? That's hard to answer. Because she did so many amazing things. So many miracles. So many acts of love. How do I pick just one?

Was it when she brought me my medication bag without being trained? Was it when she licked my wounds and helped them heal faster? Was it when she woke me from nightmares and saved me from spiritual attacks? Was it when she forced me to walk every day, no matter the weather, keeping me healthy and active? Was it when she gripped my leg as they took her away, showing me one last time how much she loved me?

All of those things were amazing. All of those things were miracles. All of those things proved she was special. Sent by God. An angel. But if I had to pick the most amazing thing? It would be that she was a part of our lives and loved us unconditionally.

She didn't judge me for having lupus. Didn't care that I was sick. Didn't leave when things got hard. Didn't complain when I couldn't play with her. Didn't resent me when I was in pain. She just loved me. Unconditionally. Completely. Every single day. For sixteen years.

She loved me when I was crying. When I was angry. When I was depressed. When I was hopeless. When I was in too much pain to move. When I couldn't walk her. When I couldn't feed her. When I couldn't give her what she needed. She still loved me. Still stayed by my side. Still licked my face. Still brought me comfort. Still reminded me: You're not alone. I'm here. I love you. And I always will.

That kind of love? That's rare. That's special. That's divine. Humans struggle to love like that. We love conditionally. We love when it's easy. We love when we get something back. We love when it benefits us. But Brown Sugar? She loved purely. Selflessly. Unconditionally. The way God loves. The way angels love. The way we should all love but rarely do.

And that love saved my life. Not just physically. But emotionally. Spiritually. Mentally. When I wanted to give up, when I thought: What's the point? Why keep fighting? Brown Sugar gave me a reason. Her love gave me a reason. Her presence gave me a reason. She needed me. And I needed her. And that was enough. That kept me going. That kept me alive.

The most amazing thing Brown Sugar ever did was be a part of our lives and love us unconditionally. That's her legacy. That's her gift. That's what I'll remember forever. Not just the miracles. Not just the healing. But the love. Pure. Unconditional. Eternal. Love.

Thank you, Brown Sugar. For sixteen years. For everything. For being my angel. For healing me. For loving me. I miss you. Every day. And I'll love you forever. Until we meet again. In heaven. Where there's no more pain. No more lupus. No more suffering. Just love. Just peace. Just you and me. Together again. That's what I'm living for. That's what I'm fighting for. To see you again. My angel. My healer. My Brown Sugar. Rest in peace, baby girl. I love you.

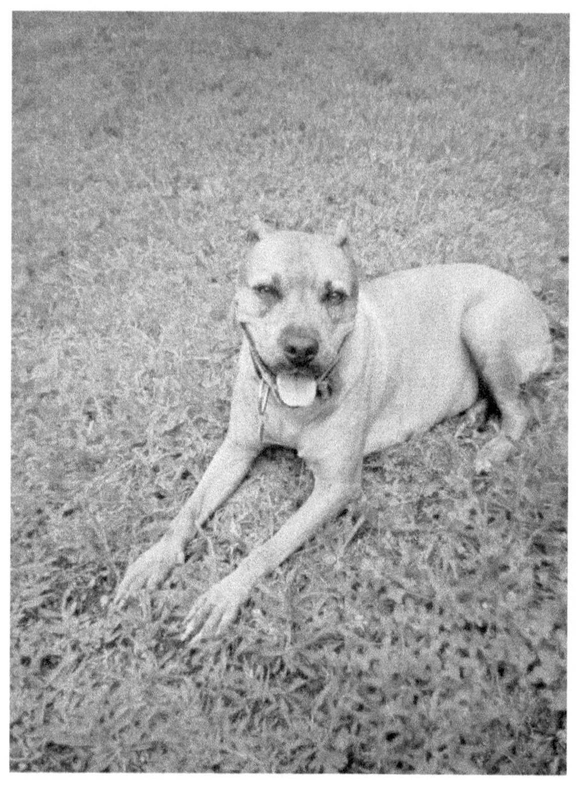

Chapter 19
The Amazing Effects of Having That Special One in Your Life

During the time earlier in my life when discovering I had lupus, around three years into trying to learn how to treat it, I always wondered would I be able to find someone special to go through it with me.

I mean would I be blessed with someone strong enough to even want to deal with watching me day and night go through the moments of the lupus taking over my body, with its side effects like joint pain, headaches, stomachaches, scars, snappy attitudes because of different mood swings, all from being in so much pain, especially when I can't even get out of bed on sometimes, when that special one really needs me?

I was always wondering would I be blessed with someone who can cope with most of the hardest struggles dealing with lupus' up and down moments.

And one day out on a beautiful Saturday night in the city of NYC, hanging out in Manhattan on my way to a club, I ran into a group of individuals who also were hanging out that night.

And yes, out of that group, that one caught my attention.

Let me tell you about that night. The night I met my fiancée. The night God put her in my path. The night everything changed.

It was a beautiful Saturday night in Manhattan. Summer. Warm. The city was alive. People everywhere. Music playing from cars. Laughter. Energy. And I was out with my friends. Dressed up. Feeling good. Wearing a powder blue jean suit with red Timberland boots. Yeah, I know. Red Timberlands. But I liked them. Thought they looked good. Thought they made me stand out.

We were heading to a club called The Speed. And as we were walking, I saw this group of women hanging out near the club. And one of them caught my eye. Stopped me in my tracks. She was beautiful. Had this presence. This energy. And I thought: I have to talk to her. I have to at least try.

So I approached her. Confident. Smiling. And I said: "Hi."

And she said: "Hi," back.

And I said: "Can I talk to you for a minute please?"

And she said: "No."

Just like that. No. Straight rejection. Didn't even hesitate.

And I was shocked. I said: "Oh wow. Word up. You're dissing me?"

And one of her friends, the one standing next to her, she laughed. And she said to my future fiancée: "Go ahead and go talk to him. He seems cool." And then she looked at my boots and laughed. "Even with those red boots."

And I said: "Y'all got jokes."

But my future fiancée still said no. Still turned me down. And I thought: Maybe it's the boots. Maybe the powder blue jean suit and red Timberlands is too much. Maybe I'm trying too hard.

So I went about my business. Went to the club with my friends. Tried to forget about her. But I couldn't. She stayed on my mind. That face. That smile. That confidence to turn me down without even thinking about it.

And after I left the club, guess what? I ran back into the same group of friends hanging out together again. And she was there. And I thought: You know what? I'm going to give it another shot. What do I have to lose? She already said no once. Can't get worse than that.

So I approached her again. And this time, she was by herself. Her friends had left. They caught the train home. And she was just walking them to the train station. And now she was heading to catch her own train.

And I said: "Hey, what's up. Where are your friends?"

And she said: "They caught the train home. I was just walking them to the train station. Now I'm going to catch the train to my home."

And I said: "By yourself?"

And she said: "Yes."

And I said: "Can I walk with you? To make sure you get to the train station safe? It's late."

And she looked at me. Studied me. Decided. And she said: "Yes."

And we walked. And we talked. And it was easy. Natural. Like we'd known each other for years. Like we were supposed to meet that night. Like God orchestrated the whole thing. The rejection. The friends leaving. The second chance. All of it.

And by the time we got to the train station, I knew: This is someone special. This is someone I want to get to know. This is someone who might be the one.

And we exchanged phone numbers. And I kept that number. On a little raggedy piece of paper. Balled up in the corner of my pocket of the same blue jean jacket I was wearing that night. And I never threw it away. Never lost it. Even though I didn't call for a long time. I kept it.

My fiancée's name is D Brown. And we have been engaged for a few years now.

And we went on a few dates after that night. And things were good. Really good. We connected. We laughed. We enjoyed each other's company. And I started to think: Maybe this could be something. Maybe this could be serious.

But then I got scared.

Why did I disappear for two years? What was I afraid of?

Commitment at that time. I had just gotten out of a relationship. I needed time to get my life back in order. And I didn't know if she wanted to be in a relationship.

Because every time I used to ask her, "Are you ready to go steady?" she'd say: "No. I just want to be friends."

So I didn't really know what she really wanted to do. And I was confused. And I was still dealing with unfinished business with my ex-girlfriend. And I was dealing with lupus. Trying to figure out how to manage it. Trying to figure out if I even wanted to bring someone new into this mess. Into this pain. Into this uncertainty.

So I stepped away from her. And it ended up being two years. Two whole years. Because I was scared. Scared of getting hurt. Scared of hurting her. Scared of commitment. Scared of lupus ruining another relationship before it even started.

But I never forgot about her. Never stopped thinking about her. And I kept that phone number. On that little raggedy piece of paper. In the corner of my pocket. Like a reminder. Like hope. Like God telling me: She's still there. When you're ready.

And one day, after two years, I decided: I'm ready. I'm going to call her. I'm going to take a chance. And if she changed her number, she changed her number. If she moved on, she moved on. But I have to try.

So I called. And she answered. And I couldn't believe it. Same number. After two years. She kept the same number.

And we were both so surprised and couldn't believe that we were on the phone talking like we never parted with each other.

And she told me later: The same day I called, she was on the phone with the same friend who told her to give me a chance that night in Manhattan. And her friend was asking her: "Whatever happened to that friend you met in Manhattan that night?" And she said: "I don't know. He just disappeared. In thin air."

And then, that same day, I called. Out of nowhere. After two years. And her friend was probably kind of shocked also after she heard that the same day they mentioned me, I called.

And after talking on the phone for a couple of days, something was on both our minds. Yes, it was funny and shocking. I was low on money one day and she loaned me a couple dollars. But I never got to give it back to her because of me straying away for those years.

So I guess you know she brought it up during one of our conversations on the phone. And yes, she demanded I bring it to her all the way in Brooklyn and I was in Jersey.

The thing I definitely didn't want to hear was that she was involved with someone for some years now from the time I wasn't around. I kind of felt really depressed a little. But I know people must move on with their lives. Because time doesn't stop for no one.

So we set up a date and I brought her her money back with interest. And we still decided to talk on the phone as friends. And I definitely tried to keep in touch. It became a weekend thing where we would only call each other. And we would talk on the phone for a good while.

So one day she didn't sound too good on the phone. She sounded down. And I asked her what was wrong. And she told me that her and the guy she was involved with had separated.

I know it's not nice to be happy to hear that type of news for anyone. But because she was special to me, I definitely was kind of happy.

So I started to plan the day I would just spill all the beans about what was going on with me. And I mean everything. So she wouldn't get caught by any surprises and get in shock.

So now that she knows everything, I'll let it be up to her to make the decision on if she wants to deal with someone like me that is in this type of position.

The first time I told my fiancée I had lupus was six months into the relationship. The second time around. After we reconnected. After we started dating seriously.

We had a conversation about why I was always kind of sick. And how did my legs get like this with all these problems.

And I said: "Well if I tell you, please don't feel sorry for me or treat me like a charity case."

So she said: "No I will never do that. So what's up, why are you always in pain? I see you work out hard every day. And sometimes it looks like it's paying off because you are full of energy. And some days you look to be down. And why are those wounds on your legs taking so damn long to close?"

So I said: "If you're getting upset and impatient with me, I'm just going to not tell you and just leave it alone.

And if you want we can just go our separate ways. Because I don't want you feeling uncomfortable about what's going on with me. This is my problem."

So she said: "I am telling you and asking you about your situation because I dealt with a similar situation."

So I said: "Yeah, well I'm suffering from lupus. You know someone who had it or who has it?"

She said: "No. What is that? How do you catch it?"

I said: "You don't catch it. You can't catch it. It's not contagious. You inherit it from a family member on either your father or your mother's side of the family. In my case it came from my father's side. My oldest auntie has it."

So she said: "So how do you get rid of it?"

I said: "You can't. There's no cure for it. It's only treatable. You can only maintain it and keep it stable and under control so you won't suffer as much with pain."

She said: "Wow."

I said: "Now see, don't say that. It's like you're so amazed that you never heard of someone suffering with a chronic disease before."

She said: "No, no. Didn't say it for that reason."

So I said: "Why you say it then?"

She said: "I said wow because if you had not said what it was and all the side effects it brings to your body, I couldn't tell it was that serious with you."

So I said: "Well don't start worrying about it. Because it's my lupus. My problem. Okay please."

She said: "Yeah but I want to help when I can. I want to help you keep it under control."

I said: "No problem. But I am not asking you or begging you. And you don't have to go spreading the news about my health situation to your family and friends please. I'd appreciate it."

So she said: "Yes, it's no one's business. I don't put no one in my private life."

So I said: "Word that's good. Because I am also a private person. I just don't trust too many people. And I cut a lot of people out of my life because they crossed me in so many bad ways. So yes, got rid of all the leeches and headaches with people who don't mean me any good in life. Case closed."

So she said: "Yeah I hear you."

So I said: "I am so glad we had this conversation."

She said: "Yeah why?"

I said: "It's been on my mind about telling you for a long time. But didn't know how you would react about it. So yeah, this is a big weight off my back and mind. Thank God you understand."

She said: "No problem."

And I felt relief. Real relief. Like I could breathe again. Like I didn't have to hide anymore. Like I could be myself. Fully. Completely. Without fear of rejection. Without fear of judgment. Without fear of her running away.

She claimed she could handle it. She's been through something similar to this type of situation with her mom at a really young age.

So now I started to feel so much more comfortable sharing my life story, my challenges I was dealing with in my life.

But even though I felt so much better getting it off my chest, and she kept saying don't worry about nothing I'll stick by you no matter what, I can handle it, I still had my doubts about how long she would hang in there with me. How long would she stick by me.

Still I was counting days, counting months, to years. I couldn't believe she hung by my side all these years, dealing with me and my lupus.

Me, my lupus, her, and our dog Brown Sugar became one proud family. We became a power team that stuck through so many tough times. We all played our part in each other's lives, especially when it came to comforting each other.

So even though we got everything out in the open with what I was suffering from, one of the hardest moments in my relationship because of lupus is when she needs me to participate in special occasions or do a lot of running around when we're clothing shopping or sightseeing in Manhattan.

Especially in the summer times when the heat is in the 80s, 90s, or 100s. My lupus will definitely be active. And I have to either go and put up with the suffering because I love her, don't want to spoil her time and fun. Or I just got to stay back home and let her get with her family or friends and enjoy herself with them for that time.

So yes, that is a moment that happens a lot of times with us while dealing with lupus.

But the hardest moment? The moment that almost broke us? The moment that I thought for sure she would leave? That happened in the first year of our relationship.

I remember we were having dinner. At my place. Normal evening. Nothing special. Just us. Eating. Talking. Enjoying each other's company.

And then my vein popped. On one of my legs. Just burst. Out of nowhere. And blood started gushing out. Everywhere. Uncontrollable. Like a faucet turned on full blast.

And I lost so much blood. So fast. That I passed out. Right there. On the floor. In the middle of dinner.

And she called the ambulance. And they came in the house to put me on the stretcher. And my body was covered in my blood all the way to my chest and neck. Soaking wet. The blood just kept coming out. Wouldn't stop. Because I was on blood thinners. And that's definitely one of the deadly side effects of being on blood thinners.

So as they rushed me to the emergency room, the doctors had to cut off all my clothing to see where the blood was shooting out from.

And even though I was passed out, I started to come through a little bit to where I opened my eyes a little bit and saw the expression on her face.

And I was so hurt. Because now she's seeing just how serious this situation is with lupus. This isn't just joint pain. This isn't just fatigue. This isn't just bad days. This is life-threatening. This is emergency rooms. This is blood everywhere. This is me passing out. This is real. This is dangerous.

So as they got me situated and cleaned up, they had to give me a blood transfusion. And when she saw this, it was another expression on her face.

I felt hurt thinking she's not going to be able to handle this type of lifestyle.

So once I got back home, we talked about it. And I just told her: "Please let's just be friends and go find someone who you don't got to go through with something like this. Please please please."

She refused to listen. She said no. She said she's staying. She said she can handle it. She said she's not going anywhere.

And I started to cry. And kept saying to myself: Who is this young woman? Where did she get this courage from? Where did she get the heart to deal with someone like me to be living with this type of health issues?

Is it because she likes my cooking? I make sure I feed her breakfast, lunch, and dinner with love. I thought I can throw in that joke because I am always teasing her about that.

But what could it be? And God spoke to me spiritually right away. I heard a voice in my head saying: Who else can it be but an angel sent from God to help watch over you, like you will watch and protect her.

No matter what her friends might have said, and I am quite sure some people in her family said that she doesn't need to be with someone like me. I know this because in the heat of a moment she will say it. But she still stuck it out with me no matter what was said.

We both believe God put us in each other's lives at the right time.

Even on my side of the family and maybe some friends, I believe they said some things about her. But I never heard it in person so I really don't know. But this is normal life. Someone is always not satisfied with someone's relationship. Especially when a couple is trying to be supportive with one another. Especially when a couple who can hang out like friends and a couple at the same time, letting people who are minding our business know that well they really must enjoy each other's company. They must really have a lot of fun. The chemistry must be strong.

So yeah, a lot of that can be going on with individuals who's not for us, I figured. I really don't see a problem with a couple hanging out as friends as well as a couple sometimes. It keeps things strong in a relationship. Also spicy. And interested in each other.

It's not just a moment or a time she was very supportive. She is always and has been very supportive with my situations living with lupus and its active side effects.

What does she do that helps me most when I'm having a bad day? Well let me tell you. She helps me cope with bad days with a good uplifting conversation. And of course, scriptures from the Bible. And she really goes deep with it. She helps out a lot when I am having a bad day.

She knows exactly what to say. Exactly what scripture to pull. Exactly what prayer to pray. And it's not surface level. It's not generic. It's specific. It's powerful. It's anointed. Like she's speaking directly to my situation. Like God is using her to minister to me. To encourage me. To remind me: You're not alone. You're not forgotten. You're not abandoned. God is with you. I'm with you. We're going to get through this together.

And that helps more than any medication. More than any doctor's appointment. More than any treatment. Because it feeds my spirit. It strengthens my soul. It gives me hope when I feel hopeless. It gives me peace when I feel anxious. It gives me strength when I feel weak.

When she sees I am not feeling good or if I am in pain, we both will respect each other. Let's just wait until we are both feeling up to the point where we can both be at our best when we want to be snuggled up with each other.

And that's important. That respect. That understanding. That patience. Because lupus doesn't just affect my body physically. It affects everything. It affects closeness. It affects that part of a relationship that's supposed to be natural and easy and spontaneous. But with lupus, nothing is spontaneous. Everything has to be planned. Everything has to be timed. Everything depends on how I'm feeling that day.

And she gets it. She doesn't pressure me. She doesn't make me feel guilty. She doesn't make me feel less than. She just waits. She respects. She adjusts. And when I'm ready, when I'm feeling good, when the pain is manageable, then we connect. Then we're intimate. Then we're close. And it's worth the wait. Because there's no pressure. No guilt. No shame. Just love. Just patience. Just understanding.

What advice would I give someone that's in a relationship and living with a chronic illness?

Well, I will tell them this. If you have someone who's trying to be in your life and you both know you will make a good future together, everything about you and each other matches up well, whatever part in your chronic disease you must play to keep it intact and stable enough to control, to feel and perform as normal as possible, you go the extra mile every time.

So the person you love can help you go the extra extra mile with you in dealing with your chronic illness together. No matter how uncomfortable you may feel some days and times. Because you know with the chronic illness you can never be 100 percent healthy and feeling well. So you have to push yourself to keep fighting not just for yourself, but for the one you love that's trying to be there to the end.

That's the advice I believe everyone who's dealing with some type of chronic illness needs to hear.

Because here's the truth: living with a chronic illness is hard. On you. On your partner. On your relationship. It tests you. It challenges you. It pushes you to your limits. And sometimes beyond your limits.

But if you have someone who's willing to stay, who's willing to fight with you, who's willing to love you through the pain, through the bad days, through the hospital visits, through the flares, through all of it, then you have something special. Something rare. Something worth fighting for.

So fight for it. Do your part. Manage your illness as best as you can. Take your medications. Go to your appointments. Follow your treatment plan. Make the lifestyle changes. Do the work. Not just for yourself. But for your partner. For your relationship. For your future together.

Because your partner is doing their part. They're learning about your illness. They're adjusting their life. They're sacrificing their plans. They're giving you grace. They're giving you patience. They're giving you love. The least you can do is meet them halfway. Do everything in your power to manage your illness so you can be the best partner you can be.

And communicate. Always communicate. Tell them when you're having a bad day. Tell them when you're in pain. Tell them when you need help. Tell them when you need space. Don't hide. Don't pretend. Don't push them away. Let them in. Let them help. Let them love you. Even when it's hard. Especially when it's hard.

And remember: they chose you. They chose to stay. They chose to fight with you. They chose to love you despite the illness. Despite the challenges. Despite the uncertainty. That's not pity. That's not charity. That's love. Real love. The kind that lasts. The kind that endures. The kind that's worth everything.

So honor that love. Cherish that person. Thank God every day for sending them into your life. Because not everyone gets that blessing. Not everyone finds someone willing to walk through fire with them. And if you have that, you have something precious. Something irreplaceable. Something sent from God.

I thank God every day for D Brown. For her strength. Her courage. Her faith. Her love. Standing by my side. Through the blood. Through the pain. Through the flares. Through the hospital visits. Through the bad days. Through all of it. She stayed. She loved. She supported. She believed.

And that's why I'm still here. That's why I'm still fighting. That's why I haven't given up. Because of her. Because of us. Because of what we have together. Because of the promise we made to each other. To fight. To endure. To love. No matter what.

That's the amazing effect of having that special one in your life. Not just surviving. But thriving. Not just existing. But living. Not just enduring. But loving. Despite lupus. Despite the pain. Despite everything. Because love is stronger than illness. Love is stronger than pain. Love is stronger than lupus. And with the right person by your side, you can face anything. Overcome anything. Survive anything.

That's what D Brown taught me. That's what so many years together has shown me. That's what our relationship proves every single day. Love wins. Love endures. Love conquers all. Even lupus. Especially lupus.

And I'm blessed. So incredibly blessed. To have found her. To have kept her number on that raggedy piece of paper. To have called after two years. To have told her about lupus. To have let her in. To have let her love me. To have built this life together. This family. This partnership. This love.

That's the amazing effect of having that special one in your life. And I wouldn't trade it for anything. Not even a cure for lupus. Because loving D Brown, being loved by D Brown, fighting lupus together with D Brown, that's made me who I am today. That's made my life worth living. That's made every struggle, every pain, every bad day, worth it.

Because at the end of the day, I don't come home to lupus. I come home to love. I come home to her. I come home to us. And that makes all the difference. That makes everything bearable. That makes life beautiful. Despite everything. Because of her. Always because of her.

Thank you, D Brown. For staying. For loving. For fighting with me. For being my angel. For being my partner. For being my everything. I love you. And I always will. Lupus and all.

Chapter 20
The Poem of My Life with Lupus

So you ask me if I can tell you more about being born as a premature baby? And what complications did I have?

Well, let me start from the beginning on how that came about.

So what I was told by my mom, my father, and my other siblings, that the time my mom was pregnant with me that she wasn't really trying to have another baby. Because she already had enough kids. Too many to handle by herself. Yes, as a single parent in the 70s, it was even harder to deal with. Compared to today with all the new and latest resources and single mom programs to help them with their family.

My mom was not trying to add another child to the six other children she was already raising by herself. My mom already had two daughters and four sons.

So at them times it used to be a rumor that in the early stages of being pregnant, which is about two to three or a little close to four months, that you can have abortions.

My other siblings told me that my mom tried to have a home abortion by eating her favorite seafood. Like the fish called whiting, smothered with hot sauce.

But she ended up having me early instead. I believe a C-section had to be performed.

So about the time they got me out of my mother's womb, I was very tiny. Very small. To where she, my siblings and my father were told by the doctor: "He will not live long because of his size."

And so they kept me in the hospital to at least try to do what they can do there in St. Joseph Hospital in Paterson, New Jersey.

But within a couple days, I believe, not too sure, but I believe that it was told to my mother and father that because St. Joseph Hospital didn't have the latest hospital equipment to keep a premature infant alive long enough to work on them, they asked my mom to sign me over to St. Barnabas Hospital in the Bronx.

Because during that time in the 70s, they had the latest equipment for procedures like that.

So that's what my mom did.

So like I'm telling you again those who's reading my book, I was told this by my mom, my father, and my other siblings. That six months later, my mom got a phone call from St. Barnabas Hospital that they still have me there in the hospital and I am doing well. And if she wants to come and visit me.

Now my mom said because she didn't have a way to get to the hospital, she called my father and his oldest sister named Auntie Sophie.

So when they got to St. Barnabas Hospital, they saw how good I was doing.

And when my mom visited me in the hospital after I was there for so long, she decided she was taking me home.

And that's what they did. They brought me home.

But before bringing me home, the doctors warned them: "He might have a lot of medical issues. So don't be surprised. Because at the beginning of us keeping him alive all this time in our hospital at St. Barnabas, we had to put lots of needles in his head. He had to be connected to a lot of tubes. Like breathing tubes, feeding tubes, heart monitor and more."

My mom and siblings used to make jokes to me by saying that I was hooked up with so many tubes I looked like Frankenstein.

So yes, this is why I made it clear that I was told by my mom and dad and siblings that all this went down about me.

So some of the medical issues I used to suffer from was asthma, heavy nosebleeds and others I can't really remember.

I stood small for so long, but ended up being the tallest of my other brothers and sisters.

And how being premature affects your health throughout your life?

At the time I was growing up while still dealing with the asthma and heavy nosebleeds, I couldn't participate in heavy physical activities. Like playing baseball and football type of sports.

I couldn't be in sunny weather too long, especially when it's very hot.

I was allergic to certain fruits and foods. Strawberries would make my lips swell up. Any type of fish with dye inside would make my asthma very active and my skin would become very itchy.

So these types of premature health issues affected me until I turned about sixteen years old. And after a while, entering my young adult life of eighteen years of age, slowly but surely, I outgrew it all.

First with the asthma. Because I started to work out more seriously.

And then the heavy nosebleeds. Because of the love I have for the boxing sport, I took a lot of punches to the nose. So my nose became strong enough not to bleed so easily.

And then because I love seafood, I just had to learn what seafood didn't have dye in them. That's how I overcame these health issue and challenges.

So you ask what do I mean by lupus using different tactics to try to stop me from continuing my journey?

And what I meant by that was the different side effects it brings. Like weight gain. Risk of different infections. Thinning bones. Osteoporosis. High blood pressure.

The lupus disease itself can cause a range of symptoms including fatigue, joint pain, skin rashes, especially a butterfly-shaped rash. And it can cause serious damage to the organs like the kidneys, heart, lungs, and brain.

So like I said before, I have the most serious systemic lupus there is.

So when I catch any rashes on my face, I make a home-made face cream.

By taking a tube of 30 SPF sunscreen lotion, mixing it with Argan oil, intensive care Vaseline, fragrance-free lotion, everything itch-free. I'll mix all of these and use it as a moisturizer that lasts up to 24 hours. And it keeps the skin looking healthy.

I maintain my appearance by working out to fit the designer clothing I wear, which is more like a sportswear casual type.

I give myself warm facials with fiber cloths. It's much softer than cotton-type cloths.

I use a grapefruit face wash and an even tone face cream because of my raccoon rash around the eyes.

And I take my time doing this. So it takes me about one hour and 20 minutes max.

So this is one of the ways I keep up with my appearance and confidence with the way I look living with lupus.

Well you're asking me what do I think about if I was to go on tour in the future and tell people of the world what it's like living with lupus?

Well I will definitely consider it. Traveling the world helping people who are suffering with the same, if not similar situation in life with some form of chronic illnesses. That is one of my dreams come true someday.

I've been through many different rheumatologists. But it was only a few who were selected as the special ones.

They take their time and make sure I am doing what I am supposed to do on keeping my lupus medications up to date. They ask about how things are with myself and what I've been up to. Like what I am doing to improve my future to live a more comfortable lifestyle.

They all hold a special type effect with me.

Like my very first rheumatologist was from Ridgewood, New Jersey, by the name of Dr. Lee B. He was more like a big brother in a sort of way. He treated me well.

Then my second rheumatologist from Hospital for Special Surgery that goes by the name Dr. Dee C. She was like a true mom. She will definitely let me have it if I wasn't doing what I was supposed to do.

And what I meant by "have it," she would point her finger at me like a mom will when she's explaining something that I need to be doing.

And if I had problems from other doctors she knew of or worked with before, she would send a notation of a letter or give a phone call to explain: "You don't have to treat him in this way because he does what he is supposed to. So please don't give him a problem."

And now the rheumatologist I am involved with now goes by the name Dr. Dimondi. She's like a younger sister and a friend you will have from high school that you will keep in contact with. She's always showing me how she's very concerned about me doing what I am supposed to do.

And that's what I mean by being a special rheumatologist in my life.

And I can't forget about the entire staff of the Valley Clinic on Goffle Road. Like Mary K, Ms. Phyllis, and all the others who ever served me at the clinic. But just know they all were very good to me. And I will never forget them as long as I live.

So you ask how did I find Valley Health Clinic?

I was recommended by my previous rheumatologist at that time. The same way I was when meeting my new family at Valley Hospital Wound Care Department. That entire staff is amazing.

For my wound care when I first get checked in, I will take off my shoes and socks and the old wrappings and old bandages.

And the wound care nurse will inspect the wounds and clean the wounds and measure the wounds to see if it's making healing progress.

And take pictures for a before and after inspection, then rub ointment of a medication, and then put on new bandages and new leg wrappings.

Then they will set a new date for me to come back and do it all over again.

Now let me share with you the poem of my life with lupus.

I was born premature and had many problems. So the pain and suffering wasn't new to me, especially what lupus tried to do to me.

The lupus tried many tactics to try to take over my body, to my life. I guess the lupus didn't know I know how to fight.

The lupus tried to kill my confidence into believing in myself by giving me these unattractive rashes all around my face. In so many ways, I guess lupus was trying to tell me to stay in my place.

I developed my own face cream to fix that problem. I guess the lupus didn't know I've always been my own personal cosmetologist, especially when the grown women told me I was handsome.

The lupus tried to cripple me by giving me varicose veins, causing my legs to swell and develop scars. But my mind was too strong, making me refuse to sit down and cry. I guess lupus didn't know I was born a warrior.

Lupus tried to steal my joy every time I tried to enjoy myself with family and friends by giving me arthritis all through my body, especially my hands. I guess lupus didn't know I'll fight it to the end.

The lupus keeps coming with it all, and I keep throwing the ball, striking it out.

I said to the lupus: "Instead of you keep trying to take me out, let's become family and go out on tour. Spread the word around the world. We don't have to be enemies since we will be living together, sharing our lives together. Let's both get strong and try to live forever. Because as a team, we will only get better. So let's just become one love and share the love to all the others who's suffering from any other disease they will have to live with for the rest of their lives."

And I want to thank all my heroes. Like my first rheumatologist to my wonderful rheumatologist of today to the whole staff of Valley Clinic Wound Care who are the best at what they do. They truly care.

I would like for readers to take into consideration of others who are really going through depressed and stressful times with pain and suffering of all types and different types and styles of chronic pain and illnesses.

So when it comes to a doctor of any kind or an ordinary healthy individual, if someone tells you that they have difficult times in life living with these health issues, just living with a chronic disease, treat them with some type of comfort and as a decent human being.

Not to be rough and act like "it is what it is, whatever."

Because people who are living with an illness of any kind who get treated wrongfully will never open up about what is going on in their lives or about how they're feeling.

Most of us living with some form of illness wouldn't even go to the doctors because we're afraid you will judge us or we might get treated roughly.

So I'm not saying treat us like a charity case. But treat us like any other individuals with respect and in a professional manner.

We are still human with feelings.

God just blessed us with a little extra life responsibility, like health issues.

And no one is exempt.

This can be your mom and dad, or even your brother or sister. And even the new life you bring into this world.

You wouldn't like to be treated wrongfully on no levels, especially when in need of help to get and become healthy again.

And for all the individuals who are suffering from systemic lupus and other forms of illnesses, stay in the fight for a better life no matter what situations you're in.

They said I wouldn't live past my first day. That I was too small. Too weak. Too premature to survive.

They hooked me up to machines. Put needles in my head. Connected me to tubes. Made me look like Frankenstein, my family said.

They were ready to give me up for adoption. Didn't think I was worth keeping. Didn't think I would make it.

And I lived.

I outgrew the asthma. Outgrew the nosebleeds. Outgrew the allergies. Became the tallest in my family. Became a boxer. Became a fighter. Became a survivor.

And then lupus came.

And lupus said: "I'll finish what being premature started. I'll take you down. I'll break you. I'll win."

But lupus didn't know. Didn't know I was born fighting. Didn't know I've been defying death since day one. Didn't know I'm still here for a reason.

So I fight. Every day. Every flare. Every pain. Every rash. Every wound. Every doubt. Every fear.

I fight with my homemade face cream. With my wound care appointments. With my rheumatologists who care. With my fiancée who stayed. With my faith that sustains. With my will that refuses to break.

I fight because I'm still here. Still standing. Still loving. Still dreaming. Still believing.

Still teaching others how to fight too.

That's my story. That's my testimony. That's my poem. That's my life with lupus.

From Frankenstein baby to lupus warrior. From tubes in my head to wrappings on my legs. From too small to survive to too strong to quit.

This is who I am. This is what lupus made me become. This is what God always knew I could be.

A fighter. A survivor. A voice. A hope.

For everyone who's fighting something nobody can see. For everyone who's been told they won't make it. For everyone who refuses to give up.

Stay in the fight. Keep going. You're stronger than you know. You're here for a reason.

Just like me.

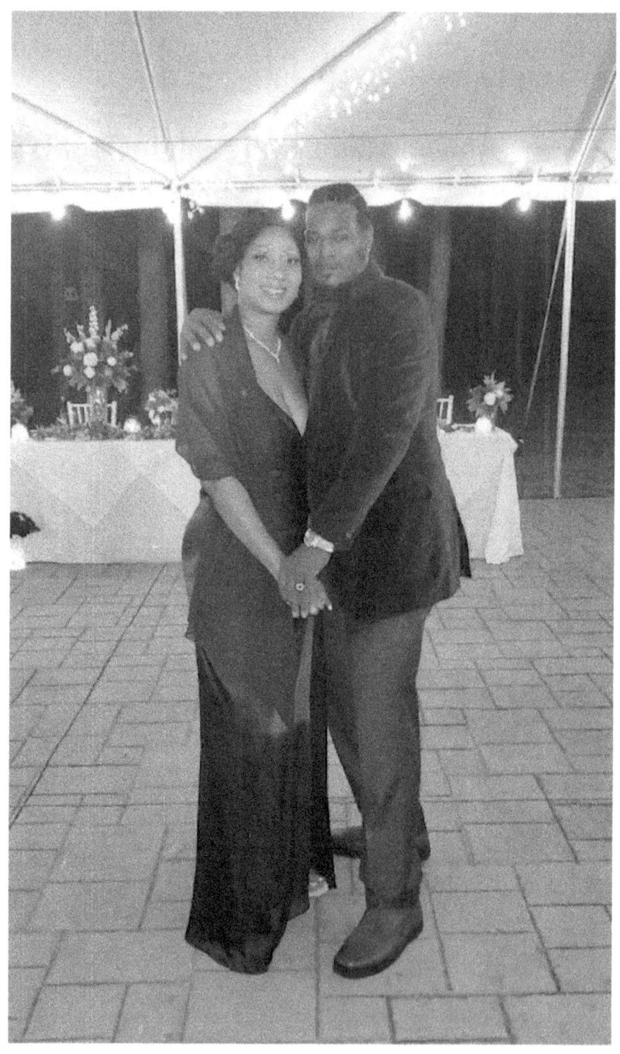

(Johnny and his Partner)

www.ingramcontent.com/pod-product-compliance
Lightning Source LLC
Chambersburg PA
CBHW070743160726
48004CB00001B/23